Tao and Diet

Promoting Health, Wellbeing and Long Life

Dongyang

ISBN:1543298249
ISBN-13: 978-1543298246

Today, technology and living standards have improved more than ever before, but people's health has sharply declined. Elderly diseases such as high blood pressure and diabetes now happen to young people. Cancer and other malignant diseases are wide spread. All of these are because the quality of our life has deviated from the concept of healthy living. This book titled "Tao and Diet" describes the relationship between Tao and food from a Taoist perspective. It is dedicated to those who are seriously care about their quality of life. It encourages the reader to use natural diet conditioning to achieve the goal of health and longevity.

Dongyang

Preface

The world has entered the new age of commercialisation, a combination of the second industrialisation and an information era when people's lives changed. It has brought about unprecedented challenge and crises in the world. This so called crisis is a result of the main media over exaggerating the benefit it has brought to the people, and this is a great misguided perception society holds. As a result people have completely ignored the existence of media harm. It has weakened people's awareness pertaining to the nuisance of new technology products. It makes people fall into a state of sickness, with their lives no longer simple and natural. Therefore, I think it is necessary to write this book about Tao and Diet. The purpose is to awaken those who are still deceived by mainstream media, to change the status quo and to maximise benefit for people's lives.

Throughout history, in addition to the nuisance that the world's industrial development has brought upon us, such as unlimited indiscriminate deforestation of natural resources, pollution of mountains, rivers, lakes and atmosphere, and industrial emissions upon the earth, the most serious matter is the issue of food safety. In order to achieve maximum interest, food production companies at the discretion of public health are sacrificing the well being of people and even costing their lives. The immoral actions such as frequent issues surrounding infant formula in the recent world, the scandal of selling contaminated horsemeat as beef, and the leanness-enhancing agent problem are just typical examples. These issues already threaten the health and survival of humanity itself.

For the purpose of obtaining a better living environment, human beings have invented and developed science and technology. The new science and technology is supposed to serve the survival of humanity with well-being as the prerequisite, but unfortunately, it all went wrong due to companies' interest driven by current development. We cannot naively expect these companies will suddenly develop a conscience and be repentant. However, each of us has the right and obligation to boycott and oppose those food production companies and enterprises that threaten the people's health. Therefore, the more people who are awakened to push forward the campaign of food safety can together make change.

Taibai Mountain*1 Taoist hermit Sun Simiao*2 accounted: *"All diseases and sudden death that occurs in mid life is mostly caused from the diet. The risk of diet is more than sensual. Sensual can be easily abandoned, but the meal cannot be skipped even once. The more benefit it is to people, the more harm it has if people get it* *wrong. Although tasty and pleasurable to eat, certain foods may conflict with each other, if the taboo of food harmony is broken, it will fall heavily to poison. In any case, people get sick after the wrong diet accumulates over years; in worse case, death by food poisoning."*

The risk of diet referred to by ancients is completely different to the risk of diet nowadays. There were no biochemical pollutions such as pesticides and chemical fertilisers, neither were there poisonous hazards such as genetically modified organism (GMO) technology in ancients' diet. There was even no integrated pollution caused by various other chemical additives and preservatives in ancient time. But the threat of food safety we are facing today is unprecedented because people have lost their behavior of self-realisation and self-restriction.

A shock wave of commercialisation has degraded the human mind/spirit of natural perception. People are blindly looking for another way to liberate themselves, trying to create a new 'reconstruction of the universe era' by using 'scientific' ways above natural law. Little do they know, cosmic forces of the infinite universe nature, has not enough time for humans to seek a new possibility. Humans will most likely be destroyed before they find a new way out. Thus, we have to get rid of the daydreaming; we have to be in harmony with nature and develop a broad path relying on Mother Nature. Only in this way can human beings meet halfway, avoid being destroyed and go on living forever.

Instead of 'no development' and 'undeveloped' problems humanity has faced in the past, the mental illness humans suffer from today is blindly advancing. Excessive growth and reckless development has occurred due to humans being too greedy. Physical weakness has indeed been caused by overwork; however the resulting illness has led people to embark on a dead-end. What takes people to the point of no return is mental illness. Mental illness creates all kinds of illness, the Qi*[3] creates all kinds of illness/diseases, and bad habits create all kind of illness.

Lao Tzu said: "*People get sick all because of wicked behaviors even though they are covered up. Some illnesses are caused by improper diet and unusual weather. Violations committed to the positive spirit of nature will cause death. It was the sage although in the dark, dared to commit crime; although with meritorious and wealth, dared to target profit. Measured the size to make one's clothes accurately; made right the amount of food to eat. Never have unbridled desire although rich and elegant; never break the law although poor and humble. If no cruelty to others, there were never sufferers of illnesses. Should it be inadvertent?*"

We all have nature, but the organs decide the human nature. The disharmony and imbalance of Yin*[4] and Yang*[5] in viscera can lead to deviations of customary mind, which results in mental illness. This needs to be kept in check if any exception in self-lifestyle or everyday living is observed. To identify the root cause and correct the deviation, a change in Mind habit is required. With perseverance you can always maintain, no problem. The illness is only can be cured through taming the unsettled mind and correcting habits to live in safety. Mental illness needs mental medicine to cure. The choice of medication is futile. This book discusses dietary adjustments that can solve this problem.

In addition, the title of the book contains the word 'Tao', which means this book is closely linked with Taoism. According to my intention, this is an article written for the guidance of internal alchemy practice, taking into account the needs of different audiences and finally focusing on the relationship between Diet and Tao. Due to the common goal of the general public to achieve both mental and physical health to reach longevity, the intention of the book is to cover all aspects of social life, so the title of the book will naturally be interpreted as "the way of eating". This book can provide some reference and guidance to people's daily lives, if only to make more people understand what a healthy lifestyle is and what a positive role a healthy diet brings.

By Dongyanzi
February 28, 2015

Dongyang

A special thank to Penelope Ford, my student, who helped me in editing to make this book published.

A special thank to Wei Liu who was in charge of the book cover design and organised all contents in this book.

CONTENTS

Dongyang

The relationship of diet, health and Tao cultivation

An important issue often overlooked when practicing internal alchemy is the adjustment of daily diet and taboos. This adjustment for people who practice is essential to avoid contraindications. The diet in this book refers to following the order of nature in accordance with changing seasons of Yin and Yang, namely by adjusting the diet to achieve best results of Yin and Yang balance of nutrients in the body.

In this vast universe, any planet should have the same opportunity as the earth, to have the same atmosphere as the earth and rotate around the star at the same time. This would enable access to the same basic conditions suitable for biological survival so life can be created. Since humans begun, sages were able to recognise the activities of human life as being closely connected to nature. The essential life is from the Yin and Yang of heaven and earth. Yin and Yang are linked to each other through integration and evolution by the five elements*6 of metal, wood, water, fire, and earth. The constant movement in this cycle derived six disadvantaged weather extremes, which are three Yin-Qi*7 of wet, dry, cold and three Yang-Qi*8 of wind, heat, fire. If people are not good at taking care of their health, they are often in violation of these five elements in nature, and disadvantaged by the changing patterns of these six weather extremes, resulting in evil energy (negative energy) bringing harm to the human body. Therefore, the ability to carry out health variation according to the balance of Yin and Yang is essential to achieve health and longevity.

From above we know humans are connected to the weather. That is to say if the Yang-Qi in the human body is as clear as the weather, it can make people's mood calm and emotions stable. If such conditions are met, Yang-Qi can be sufficient enough to play a role in protecting the human body. Even if attacked by deceitful wind and evil energy, the body will not be harmed. People who are good in maintaining health can always keep the body's Yin and Yang circulating and in harmony with external Yin and Yang. Therefore the Mind can be recuperated and never slackened to suit the weather change. On the contrary, people who are not good at maintaining health will make protective Qi in the body lax, and the Qi of nine apertures of the human body will be blocked, the Qi of muscle will be obstructed, sluggish and adverse. The resistance of disease will be greatly reduced. This is entirely due to Yang-Qi being greatly weakened by one's own negligence. Understand the importance of Yin and Yang in maintaining health and adjust the diet according to the secret rules of Yin and

Yang.

Although the aim of this book is to inform dietary requirements related to Taoist cultivation, ordinary people can use this knowledge to empower themselves and I believe receive promising results too.

We often say illness enters by the mouth; trouble comes out by the mouth. This sentence tells the plain truth of the reality of our society, but is easily ignored. Careless or extreme diets are definitely harmful to the body, but if the right way of diet is mastered, illness will not enter by the mouth. Therefore, we should spare no effort to do the task of diet well. We must not damage ourselves and have lifelong regrets due to not treating with right remedies.

This book is titled Tao and Diet. It actually means the way of diet. Since it is the Tao, it is completely different from secular diet. The difference herein is, all the food and drink are related and matched with Tao. So instead of the ordinary fate of humankind, people can enjoy a healthy and happy life in all directions. The original intention of this book was to help internal alchemy practitioners achieve the right way of diet, however it now accounts for the wishes of both Taoism enthusiasts and ordinary people looking for a better, healthier life. More and more people are taking action to avoid worry and risk so they can achieve greater success in business and enjoy a better life.

The impact of environment, climate and diet on human health

As mentioned in the previous chapter, to follow natural order, the diet should be adjusted in accordance with Yin and Yang changes in season. Furthermore, to follow these changes of spring, summer, autumn and winter, is to follow external climatic changes of cold, heat, dryness and dampness, and adjust diet accordingly. However, this adjustment differs according to each person's geographic location. Therefore it is a three-dimensional multi-faceted comprehensive adjustment mechanism.

Giving an example, the temperature and dampness in northern and southern extents of China are very different. People should regulate the dietary content based on their geographical location. People who live in the southern humid region should always drink red bean and barley soup to eliminate body moisture and prevent the intrusion of rheumatism. For Northerners it is precisely the opposite. The northern winter is cold and dry and people tend to use the heater or heating, thus increasing the hazards of dryness. Therefore people should take extra care to eat more Yin foods such as lotus root, turnip, etc., to confront dry weather from the inside.

In addition, the natural environment influences the physique from generation to generation, of people living in the south compared to people living in the north. The recent migration of these people to the new environment has caused two different results either: slow adaptation to the new environment or succumb to a variety of illnesses. Although there is a third kind of person interposed between the two who adapts with slight adverse reaction while their overall health and life are not affected. This applies to people who live in the regular world.

The different physical condition of the human body comes from living in different regions and climate. Chinese people in the northwest eat more beef and lamb so they are likely to suffer from high cholesterol. The diet of people in northeast alpine areas is rather salty so they are likely to suffer from the internal heat or internal cold. Southern area is humid and hot, so people who live there are likely to suffer from spleen and/or stomach diseases. Different climatic regions also affect crops. Sanya in Hainan province of China belongs to subtropical climate. It is warm all year round and plant growth is very vigorous. The incessant growth of the plants has resulted in excessive loss of soil nutrients. Plants cannot absorb adequate nutrients from the soil, so the taste of cucumbers, corn and rice in that area is bland.

If you decide to cultivate the Tao quietly and crave success in the future, then you should be strict with diet discipline. It is not necessary to abstain from meat exactly like the temple monks, neither is it necessary to eat meat every meal. The right choice is to arrange in pairs the meat and vegetables strictly and correctly to meet practice requirements in the secular world. People who live in the social world cannot avoid interacting with others. Behavior based on reciprocity, intertwined drinking in large groups and excessive intake of meats all bring unnecessary damage to the human. Therefore, we need a clear understanding and certain assurance of diet to control food intake strictly. The Taoist classic book, Yellow Court Canon states: "The fruit of all grains is the essence of the land. It can produce tasty flavors; it can also produce disgusting smell and stink to disrupt the consumer's mind and positive spirit and damage people's original Qi, the vital essence of life. How can you rejuvenate with this?"

Daily dietary intake must be in accordance with the principle of nutritional balance. We must understand well the difference of diet in distinction throughout the ages to make adjustment accordingly based on different gender, with particular attention to light food and paired arrangements of meat and vegetables. As physical and daily activity is greater in young adults compared with old people, their rate of consumption is certainly larger. More meat than vegetables can be considered when arranging their daily diet. The elderly because of their weaker digestion and absorption systems, coupled with fewer activities, should appropriately reduce the intake of meat to avoid variety of diseases caused by indigestive toxins accumulated in the body. In addition, the man's body type belongs to Yang and easily he suffers from excessive heat so the man should try to reduce baked or fried high-protein food. Woman's body type belongs to Yin, high protein foods can nourish Yin to bring up Yang so she can probably eat more heat type foods.

The most typical hazard of an improper diet is firstly encountered as a variety of tumors and cancer; the second is fatal blood disease such as heart disease, hypertension, brain hemorrhage, stroke and so on, which collectively named as cardiovascular and cerebrovascular diseases. To avoid entanglement with hazards associated with these diseases, prevention becomes extremely important as the approach in daily life, and ordinary daily routine becomes the key factor to access health and longevity. Routine precautions become the knowhow on eating healthy, disease is prevented through diet, and longevity is achieved by reconditioning the diet. The Long March begins with one step. A hundred story building rises from soil. The final achievement is all thanks to subtle accumulations. To obtain health and longevity we must rely on the benefit we receive from daily practice rather than the popular saying of "human life is determined by the God and genetics." Quanzhen practice mantra is: "my life is determined by myself rather than God," which fully reflects the Taoist concept of health.

All three meals in a day should have vegetables to supplement vitamins and fiber the right amount of meat to add protein, and the five grains as staple food to supplement various vegetarian proteins the body needs. To have five vegetables assisting five grains is just for this reason. In addition, a variety of beans are included in this context. Since some beans contain micro-toxicities, they must be cooked before eating.

Notwithstanding, most soft drinks on the market contain various chemical additives that are a health hazard and cancer risk, it is suggested to drink tea often. Tea has the benefit of cleaning the blood so ideally it should be the preferred daily health drink.

In China, there is an old saying that states: "five grain base, five sparse supplements." This is absolutely true. It straightforwardly tells what is a balanced healthy diet. The symbol of human civilisation is neither the number of artificial 'materials' created, nor the products manufactured through invention of mass production led by scientific and technological advances. The choice and cultivation of food truly embodies where the human civilisation today. The discovery and improvement of original food fully reflects the real human wisdom of our ancestors. The human survival and development has been made possible and secured over time long before the arrival of modern civilisation. Unfortunately and quite sadly, the thing is that the advent of modern civilisation interrupted and destroyed the original natural balance, and placed a terrible shadow over humanity. The people of today have completely forgotten where the human ancestors came from. The so-called Western civilisation replaced traditional lifestyle entrenched in people from the past, and dominated the whole world. People no longer take grain-based food and have tea as a healthy drink. Instead, a wide variety of chemical additives in fast food and soft drinks are everywhere. Most of these cannot be called food but man-made chemicals. Inorganic chemistry replaced natural organic food. How ridiculous and terrible this creative 'modern civilisation' is! Isn't the human destroying themselves?

The diet needed for Taoist practice to maintain good health certainly has to respect and observe the law of nature. We should take the most stringent attitude towards the daily diet because it relates to human life and the final success or failure of the practice. We should not be shirked without dishonor to resist against those who violate resolutely the natural traditional diet. Only in this way we can ensure that our lives will not be swayed by others and values of our thought will not inadvertently be modified by others imperceptibly. GMO food spreading on the market will bring an extremely serious threat to human life and reproduction so we must unequivocally oppose and resist it. The more help and convenience technology gives us today, the more harm and distress it will bring to us. The problem is, the food required in original simple daily form becomes complicated and difficult to source due to the involvement of interest groups. Driven by the great interest, the government has no choice but to make a concession for the interest groups and introduce a series of laws and regulations that bring harm to human health. For example, by not labeling GMO food and by ignoring the potential hazard of GMO food, this is elevated to the level of political and social issue.

The history tells us: As long as a country guards its own territory, all other issues are easy and simple. In other words, once the country is conquered and occupied, anything else is out of the question. If the sovereignty and territory are gone, the nation is no longer a nation; people will naturally fall to the state of slavery without any rights. This definition today is obsolete because the way of aggression against a country today has seen a fundamental and dramatic change. It no longer needs to use gunboats to open the gate of a country but just let all countries follow the same game plan, which is globalisation. If you accept the rules of their game then you have to open your market to give them freedom for dumping their naughty garbage and poisoning the consumer with genetic modified crops. It was naive to think just by not purchasing and not consuming imported genetic modified soybeans and corn products that we could avoid being poisoned. Although you can avoid direct consumption of genetic modified products, you cannot avoid eating beef, lamb and poultry etc., which the meat of livestock and poultry is fed with GMO. The result of this indirect harm is even worse than direct harm. To damage and weaken the quality of the population is an ideal way to weaken a country. Because of this, the mastermind of the country and the political interest group behind the production of these products uses this method to achieve ultimate invasion of another country to control the world on purpose. Wouldn't it be easier and more cost-effective to start a war to conquer a country? Both have the same purpose.

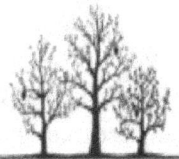

The role of the spirits in life

Alcoholic spirits are not a subjective invention by ancient tribal people, purely an accidental discovery from living. It seems to me the origin of alcohol was in fact a natural formation. The first spirit that was discovered was fruit wine. A variety of wild fruits dropped on the ground when they were ripe. Since fruit juice contains sugar, exposed and combined with the natural yeast on the peel, it fermented to wine under suitable temperatures in summer. Secondly the milk wine appeared in the same way. The milk of animals and livestock contain lactose so it can become milk wine after fermentation. Grain wine appeared rather late because the carbohydrate of the grain contains starch not sugar. Starch requires amylase to decompose sugar to brew wine. This process is much more complex than natural fruit wine, so the grain wine appeared relatively late. Despite the complexity of grain wine brewing, it is basically no different from fruit wine. At that time, since there were no way to properly store grains, the food mildew was quite common. The earliest document about food fermentation is 'Ju-Nie (鞠蘖)'. Moldy grain is called 'Ju' and activated/sprouted grain is called 'Nie'. From Chinese words you can see both contain the character '米', meaning rice. Shuo-Wen-Jie-Zi, the original Han dynasty Chinese character dictionary also defined: "Nie as rice sprout." "Rice as grain seed." Thus we know, Ju and Nie as first recorded in the literature came from sprouted and moldy grain. Later on, people started using malt (麴, pronoun Qu) instead of rice sprout. This separated the production method of Nie and Qu, and people dedicated the use of Nie for sweet wine production for ceremonies. During a thousand years from Shang dynasty (about 17th century B.C. to about 11th century B.C.) and Zhou (1046 B.C. to 249 B.C.) until the Han dynasty (202 B.C. to 8 A.D.), sweet wine from Nie was very popular.

Finds from archaeological excavations and confirmation in documents, made us fully understand the emergence of wine and how the wine was used. People used naturally fermented leftover food to produce drinkable fermented glutinous rice. Strictly speaking, it cannot be called spirits. People gradually developed a genuine process of brewing a pure grain alcoholic spirit based on glutinous rice wine. Then people slowly discovered the wine features and variety of practical effects. For instance, drinking spirits can help people warm up in cold winter; drinking or directly applying spirits to a wound can help blood circulation for injuries such as contusion, sprain or fracture from falls or blows. In fact, the first appearance of spirits was solely for the purpose of treating disease. In a controlled manner, the spirits were used to boost medicine treatment in combination with a variety of herbs known for treating a variety of diseases. Hence the saying: "spirits are the parent of all medicines". Therefore, spirits were mainly presented as medicine spirits rather than as an everyday drink in ancient people's lives. Ancient people were not like the people today who drink the spirits as juice to get drunk and consume in excess in common place.

Alcohol spirits are connected to the spirit. People in ancient times often needed to worship sky and earth so they could have the assistance of the spirits to interlink with universal spirit. That is why we say the wine has a very important function in this regard. Wine can also embolden as the folk saying states: "strong spirits counsel people guts," that is because when people drink spirits, the gall is activated so it can strengthen a man's courage. But the spirit production and brewing process of today are totally different from the method in ancient times. It makes the drinker worse off and no doubt causes great harm to people's health.

Although the alcohol brings a lot of fun and help to our lives, drinking improperly also brings a negative impact on our health, sometimes even catastrophic consequence. For this reason, we should learn the knowledge and master the method about wine drinking and treatment of disease in order to prepare for contingencies.

Often excessive drinking can lead to diabetes and high blood pressure. On the other hand, a small amount of proper spirit can certainly have a positive medicinal effect on blood circulation and metabolism for aged people in appropriate weather conditions. In a severe cold northern winter, the older people lack outdoor activities and tend to stay in a warm room all day, which can cause metabolic disorders. At this point if they can drink a little spirits often, it will have a good effect to improve blood circulation, increase metabolism and improve the immune system. Women are easily attacked by cold, which affects their Ren-Mai channel*[9], Chong-Mai channel*[10], Dai-Mai channel*[11] and liver channel and leads to stagnation. Therefore, women in childbearing age are better to drink a small glass of white wine in the night. In addition, the small Huo-luo-dan*[12] must be taken together with yellow wine. Yellow wine can smooth the channels; it can be used externally and internally. Warm yellow wine can also help as treatment for female uterine bleeding. The spirit has the power to move the blood and Qi through the blood vessels. Therefore this is the first ingredient of Chinese herbal lore and in highest position above all other medicines. Many medicines used for the treatment of gynecological diseases are inseparable from the spirits, acting as medicine booster. The spirits have a lot of effectiveness, but the spirits for treatment must be prescribed as the cure for the right disease symptomatically, and should not be taken disorderly. Likewise, the hypertension patient should not drink ginseng wine.

Excessive heat*13 caused by improper diet and its impact

Outbreaks of disease are the same as other forms of disaster characteristic of periodic episodes. This is because the accumulation of energy requires time. Other forms of disaster such as war, earthquake, flood and volcanic eruption of unusual phenomenon or natural movement also require periodic energy accumulation. Once accumulated to a certain extent, outbreak and eruption occur. It is very important to understand this natural law so we can prepare in advance to avoid or reduce damage caused by the disaster. This is the best strategy for active prevention and mitigation of disaster. This strategy also applies to the prevention and treatment of disease.

The most typical and commonly ignored disease is periodic episodes of flu. Not only for ordinary people, even among academia there is fallacious cognition. It is widely believed that a virus causes a flu outbreak. In fact it is not. According to Taoist theory, it is due to another reason. The temperature change outside is just an external factor. Without an internal factor of excessive heat inside the body, the explosion of flu cannot be driven. The accumulation of internal heat coupled with external cold, makes the lungs suddenly cold, and at high heat conditions causes an imbalance of Yin and Yang in lung mechanism, which creates stagnation of lung fluid. The intake of plenty of fluids will cause cough and shortness of breath. This is the sickness, known as the flu. The outbreak of flu every time has an adverse effect on the lungs to weaken the lungs. Every occurrence of flu the people get in their lifetime will cause cumulative damage to lungs and make lungs more fragile, eventually leading to death due to lung failure. What a terrible thing this is. We must not ignore the flu, this commonly seen 'small illness'. If you do not follow the Taoist principles of natural balance of Yin and Yang to arrange your daily diet to maintain Yin and Yang balance, you are likely to suffer from this or that disease.

For the purpose of health and longevity, I particularly draw attention to 'excessive heat' problems that have troubled us along the way. I believe most people treat excessive heat with a dismissive attitude. Some people even think that excessive heat is a common symptom and since everybody gets it there is no need to treat it seriously. There are some people who think that excessive heat only relates to small ailments and therefore not a problem since it will naturally go back to normal without treatment. There are also some people who simply take a bit of Chinese medicine to reduce the internal heat regardless of whether it is the right medicine prescribed. These attitudes and modulations are not good methods at all. In fact, the 'excessive heat' and 'promiscuous personal life' are quite similar to a country's turmoil. If a person is always in a vicious cycle in which excessive heat cannot be effectively curbed, his life will be threatened eventually. The same goes for a person who is promiscuous all the time with over-indulgence, as this will undoubtedly lead to premature aging and the disaster of suffering fatal disease. Similarly for a country, continued national unrest will lead to the decline of a nation's power and therefore the internal trouble will lead to outside aggression. China in the late Qing Dynasty is one of the most typical examples. The rise of Taiping Heavenly Kingdom greatly weakened the ruling power of the Qing government's centralisation and national strength, and ultimately led to the ruthless invasion on the Qing by Eight-Nation coalition. The troubles of ceded territory and reparations at that same time have still not completely been eliminated.

Now let's take a look to see how the excessive heat gradually leads us to the drowning disaster.

People of adolescent age most likely ignore the issue of excessive heat, because young people are full of positive energy and have nothing to worry about given their valued strong physiques. Therefore, once they suffer from excessive heat, it would be both outside heat and internal heat attacking the body simultaneously. In light cases, it would only be a soft flu with cough and running nose, followed by recuperation back to normal within a few days' of treatment. In severe cases, the symptoms would be fever, lung infection, upper respiratory tract infection and even acute pneumonia; that can in turn lead to chronic pneumonia. In this case, one cannot be recuperated with only a few days' treatment. If it cannot be treated with medication, it can lead to complications.

How do people get this 'excessive heat' ultimately? And how do we prevent it? People throughout their experiences in general social life have largely and totally ignored this. However, we can actually find answers within people's daily lives. Let's take a closer look at details of people's family lives in China and the world. We can easily see common problems and errors existing. Blindly, the parents of the children give their children too many nutritious foods such as fried meat, large amounts of dairy products and nuts to eat for their growth. These foods for teenagers easily drive excessive heat. Once or twice is not a problem, but regular consumption will make the 'heat' accumulated. This is because fish creates heat and meat creates phlegm. Plus the heat that has been stored in processed, barbecued or fried food, when ingested creates heat that will slowly be released into the stomach to grill five viscera and six bowels and make further heat to penetrate into the blood. The 'heat' that results from this will naturally burn up with inflammation, i.e. rise up to cause mouth sores and swollen eyes. If instead of striking the head, the 'heat' is retained inside the body, this will be reflected in corresponding facial features as the external indicators of organ trouble. Young people who are going through physically strong growth periods easily get excessive heat across all four seasons. Plus when parents do not even have basic knowledge of traditional life, it makes matters worse and out of control. In today's so-called civilised world dominated by the West, traditional valuable knowledge is easily abandoned resulting in people living today in a 'crisis of civilisation'. It appears sufficient scientific knowledge cannot solve the problem that needs to be solved. The issues such as social problems, health problems, diagnosis and treatment of disease, social unrest and natural disasters, etc. haunt us every day, but we do not have very effective methods and countermeasures. Just as mentioned above for the youth's 'heat', the lack of effective control will cast a shadow over their future life in light cases but ruin their future in severe cases.

Excessive heat specifically experienced in adolescence is: an excess of heat caused by a deficiency in Yin energy which is also known as substantial heat. The patient feels like they are being scorched in fire and cannot be settled. The patient comes with red face and looks ill all the time. All six vital organs fail and the mind is distraught with anxiety. Severe symptoms are shown as babbling nonsense and so on. All these greatly affect young people's daily life and learning. Attacked by both liver heat and heart heat, the mind becomes distraught with anxiety making them unable to concentrate on their studies. This results in a decline in academic performance and turns into a vicious cycle. It is not difficult to imagine future consequences with lack of proper treatment and guidance. So therefore we must take all precautions in advance to do specific work such as maintaining the daily diet of Yin and Yang. In other words to maintain the balance, grilled and fried food and meat should be paired up with steamed and stewed food and vegetables, to prevent teenagers' heat. It will kill two birds with one stone to ensure the problem of excessive heat is avoided that easily occurs at this age, while providing sufficient nutrition and delicious food.

The excessive heat is more dangerous to middle-aged adults. Why more dangerous? Because the adult is at the prime of life, and as Lao Tzu said, "the limit of maturity is heading declination." Meaning any human with material development approaching the zenith will go downhill. Should one be careless, it would be like a river with receding tide, pouring life away day by day to drive premature aging and death caused by decline and inability. The careless here means that if a small ailment or disease such as excessive heat in daily life is not prevented or modulated, it will become extremely dangerous. The threat and harm of excessive heat on middle-aged adults mainly manifests as inflammation due to excess internal heat. Also poor general health condition will cause Yin deficiencies in liver and kidney. It will bring to people symptoms including tinnitus, palpitations and sharp vision decline etc. Repeated excessive heat on gums will also bring signs of premature aging like loose or even fallen teeth. So excess of the heat is extremely dangerous and harmful to people in their prime.

If the excessive heat is more dangerous to middle-aged adults, then it is even scarier for the elderly. That is because it can be said that excessive heat reaches dangerous/ terror levels on an elderly population. This saying is not an exaggeration. Once an elderly person gets excessive heat, his whole life will be severely affected and he cannot carry on as usual. As time goes by and due to the hardship of the life, the three energies of Jing*14, Qi and Shen*15 in an elderly body are greatly reduced and not enough as when he was young. If an unexpected heat enters the body at this time, it will be extremely difficult to get rid of. The body will fall into the old and ill situation and all sorts of complications arise. Also, because the elderly are deficient in Qi and lacking liquid of the body, this means the genuine fire of kidney is no longer easily consolidated due to the weak kidney Qi. When the weather undergoes dramatic change in temperature, it will lead to inflammation whereby kidney heat is mixed with external heat. The position where the heat remains in the body will be the part experiencing discomfort and maybe even worse, where disease occurs. Giving another example, if heat attacks the midriff channel, it will cause constipation. Frequent constipation can lead to metabolic disorders from bad breath to cancerous tumor.

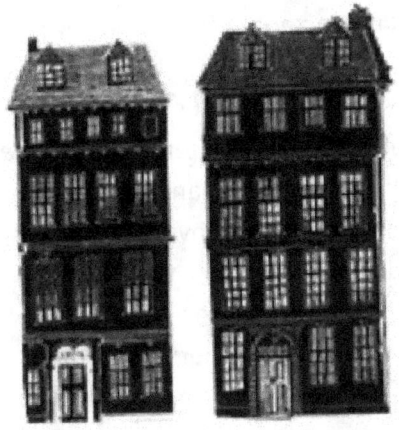

Improper diet causes vascular disease - atherosclerosis

Modern lifestyle brings us a life full of morbid age. Another often overlooked problem which affects human health is the problem of the blood's health. The most representative disease closely related to blood's health is the human killer arterial sclerosis syndrome, commonly known as atherosclerosis. If the excessive heat mentioned in the previous chapter only affected people's health in the short term, arteriosclerosis would not be a big threat to human life. Arteries play a very important role in human physiology to transfer water, oxygen and nutrition to the human body. The characteristic of arteriosclerosis presents as hardening of the blood vessel wall and narrowing of the vessel. This disease in today's society is showing an increased trend. Nobody can say he will not get arteries hardening disease in his life unless he is a real practitioner.

The terrible thing of arteriosclerosis is mainly high mortality rate. If the outbreak part of atherosclerosis is not fixed, it can occur in any part of the body. Former Yugoslav President Tito suffered from this disease, undergoing amputation caused by hardening of the arteries in the foot, and then finally lost his life due to the failure of kidney, heart and other organs. There are 87% of people aged around sixty or seventy who unfortunately suffer from arteriosclerosis. Once the hardening of the arteries happens, it is very difficult to return to normal, and there is no way like organ transplant to replace each of the vessels although we basically do not encourage organ transplants. Replacing the problem body part as you would replace a machine part cannot solve the fundamental problem.

Internal lesions of the body are due to a particular lifestyle or eating habit accumulated over a long period. It cannot be resolved by organ replacement. Western medicine simply removes or replaces the onset organ which cannot eradicate the real root cause of the disease. It is unhelpful. Today, because of the huge changes in people's life structure, a sharp increase in the incidence of cardiovascular disease has occurred and the trend is gradually rising in youth. There is concealment when the disease is light at the early stage so people cannot feel it but its harm is very destructive. The main harm is myocardial infarction, cerebral infarction and tumors. Infarction means blockage. Sometimes it cannot be identified from clinical examination. If infarction occurs in the brain it can lead to hemiplegia and/or aphasia. There are also infarctions that occur in the kidney and obstructions that occur in the large intestine. Tumor is mainly hemangioma related. Hemangioma rupture can lead to huge bleeding and death.

What kind of people are likely to suffer from atherosclerosis syndrome? The answer is actually simple. As the saying goes it is the three aged people: the aged intellectual; the aged leadership; and aged bosses. People like Churchill, Roosevelt and Stalin all died of arteriosclerosis. Since aged folk are better-off than any other age group, their diet is unrestricted, and delicious food is available at all times. This phenomenon became more common in the twenty-first century, so that on top of the three aged groups of people there is another, aged ordinary people with their specific incessant work, they are very prone to lack of physical activity and minimum exercise. To solve this problem and phenomena, there appeared such doggerel among society: "restrain your mouth, stride your legs." This simple and plain philosophy of life is more effective than all the so-called experts' talk and more practical than all the drugs.

The relationship between atherosclerosis and diet is inseparable. Simply to summarise, atherosclerosis is caused by low intake of vegetables that contain vitamins and fibre and excessive intake of meat foods that are high in fat and cholesterol. As it is often said, eating too well and moving too little are the leading cause of morbidity. Now fast foods are popular like KFC's fried chicken, McDonald's burgers and a variety of soft drinks such as Coke, Sprite and so on. 'Convenient delicious' fast food and soft drinks stimulate people's taste buds, but the use of unhealthy ingredients caused hardening of arteries for today's people from a young age. Fast food is not convenient for people's lives at all, instead a genuine death trap is prepared for people. In the past, people were at the onset of disease just after they reached old age. But now, the people who suffer from illness have changed from the elderly population to middle-aged groups. This is all because people from an early age eat too much of the food that easily causes atherosclerosis.

Internal and external factors are the two causes that eventually lead to the onset of atherosclerosis. The incidence of internal cause is counted as 20% to 30%, while external cause is counted for 70% to 80%. There are also genetic causes like family habits, such as the commonly seen family genetic history of hypertension and family genetic history of diabetes. These people must be very careful and take precaution. They must strike a balance between work and rest in life and strive as much as possible towards early prevention of the harm caused by hyperglycemia, high cholesterol, hypertension, functional hypertension, high muscle anhydride, high weight and high psychological pressure etc. Do not wait and seek medical treatment at the onset of disease. It will only lead to disappointment and suffering because people cannot receive any treatment beyond basic diagnosis after the onset of disease.

Consequences of human development and progress of

science and technology has brought extremely horrible results. Although science and technology is more developed; the people's health is more unsecure and the people's physical fitness is much worse. Since the development of various technologies, basic human physical activities have been completely replaced, resulting in less movement of muscle and body parts, making it unbearable for the basic physical burden that is needed in daily life. In the past, people always took time walking to the theater to watch a movie and home after that. How healthy it was. By the seventies and eighties televisions appeared. People no longer needed to go out and enjoy, watching instead at home what used to be at the theater. People were able to view all human stories and colorful fantasy worlds from this small screen. Then it progressed so that now almost every room has a TV. It was manual control in the beginning, and then improved to remote control, so people could easily avoid the labor of watching TV, as if sleeping in a coffin. The original walk has been replaced by a comfortable luxury car. In short, people no longer need working muscles, and have truly become idiots who never move four limbs and who cannot distinguish the five crops. The juxtaposition of the non-working body is that people eat better and better, move less and less, causing severe imbalance of metabolism. A large amount of undigested food accumulates and becomes deposited in the body, blocking blood vessels by making blood vessel walls thicker and circulatory pathways narrower. This kind of life directly leads to the outbreak of diseases.

Mortality due to various sorts and varieties of vascular disease caused by unhealthy diet and lifestyle is just less than car accident mortality rates. Today, the incidence of arteriosclerosis is ranked first among mortal diseases. The aneurysm caused by arteriosclerosis is most dangerous. Its distribution is uneven on the human body. The onset of disease is aggressive on some parts and subject to slow onset in other parts, but the harm is the same. Dissecting aortic aneurysm is also very dangerous. A quarter of people with this disease die within 15 minutes, while half of the deaths caused by this disease happen within 48 hours. Historically, Einstein died of aneurysm rupture and the American volleyball player Hyman also died of an aneurysm.

Blood vessels are throughout the body and atherosclerosis happens in the first instance. We should not loosen our prevention-oriented strategy because of rapid progress of today's medical technology. Nor blindly believe that the disease had nothing to do with our own actions and can be cured through forthcoming treatment accordingly. Yes, there are highly skilled doctor's with magical hands who can bring the dying back to life, but not everyone is lucky enough to get a skilled doctor to treat them immediately after the onset of disease and survive. Many people left the world before being rushed to hospital. Therefore, the only chance of beating the treatment of such a dangerous and deadly disease is to never wait and evaluate to resolve the problem at the point when it becomes uncertain and irremediable. Otherwise it will be too late. It is best to water the tree before it perishes and save it from drought, thus to prevent in advance. The approach to prevent the hardening of the arteries is quite simply to achieve four specific requirements: "restrain your mouth, stride your legs, take appropriate medicine, and adhere to drink plenty of water". To sum it up is to use the principle of 'food and medicine come from the same source,' make the greatest possible use of Yin and Yang of foods, correct the imbalance of Yin and Yang in the body and achieve the health. This is the way of diet; this is the real purpose of this book. To control the mouth needs to be started as early as from a child. Meat and vegetables must be paired up in the diet. Onions, garlic and tomatoes have lipid-lowering effect. These vegetables need to be eaten regularly. To 'stride your legs' is to adhere to exercise, however only everyday walking excises can achieve the prevention effect. To take appropriate medicine, is to use traditional Chinese medicine properly in accordance with body condition. It is vital the blood pressure is maintained, stabilised and controlled. Even if the blood pressure is a little high it will not matter as long as the blood pressure remains steady. Blood sugar too low is not good. Both blood sugar and blood lipids should be within the normal range. To adhere to drinking plenty of water is to transfer liquid continuously around the body to reduce blood viscosity.

It is important to be appropriate and to persevere. Long-term effort will achieve stability and balance, and ensure the best results are received.

Positive and dialectical treatment will make the therapy easy. We have entered an invasive minimalist era whereby it is easy to diagnose diseases and also easy to undergo treatment. Therefore, we must seize the opportunity as soon as possible to resolve the issue ahead of time and in time. The onset of disease happens at the beginning or at the end. Prevention of myocardial infarction is very vital. Intestinal infarction is also extremely dangerous. We cannot wait and evaluate to resolve the problem at the point when it becomes uncertain and irremediable. Otherwise it will be too late. Trees must be watered to survive from drought. People are the same.

Improper diet causes deadly disease - cancer

The disease of cancer in today's human society has already become common place. In the past, this was an extremely rare fatal illness, but today in the twenty-first century it is across every corner of the world. Currently in China, one person will be diagnosed with cancer in every six minutes. We can say that the growth and spread of cancer is closely associated with industrialisation and development of technology. Industrialisation and technology has brought a landmark progress of human civilisation, but has also had a negative impact on human reparability. The change in eating habit is one of the most typical results of industrialisation, and now all the food and drink people consume are marked with industrialisation. A variety of toxic chemical additives for various purposes have been added to the food products from the production stage of raw materials to finished products. In addition to the harm brought by the impact of industrialisation on the human body, there is also long-term damage on the human body caused by the people themselves who are too gluttonous on cold food intake to consider their god of the belly, even for a moment. People do not know that this wrong habit of diet has planted in them the root of cause of the cancer.

Human nature has its own inherent set of strict immune system traits. These are known in the West as leukocytes or macrophages. The main function is to protect the body against microorganisms outside and other antigens that may harm the human body. In fact, Taoism-t knew these secrets of the human body thousands of years earlier than Western medicine. They are named the three 'Hun's and seven 'Po's. They are actually the protection spirits of the human. Three 'Hun's are: the original positive spirit on behalf of the light of life – Taiguang; the wisdom spirit that determines a person's clever root – Shuanling; and the lust spirit that has a potential sexual orientation – Youjing. The comfort of these three spirits determines a person's well-being. So we need to continually cultivate ourselves everyday to nourish these three spirits to take better care of our lives. Seven 'Po's refer to residual information based on animal instinct that has remained in our body and consciousness. Their names are: Tunzei, Shigo, Neihui, Xiufei, Queyin, Feidu and Fushi. 'Tunzei' plays a defensive guard duty on macrophages to protect the body from enemy invasion and harassment from the outside. 'Feidu' is responsible for expelling toxins from the body, and works together with 'Tunzei' to destroy all antigens including cancer tumor cells and so on that invade the body. However, due to very popular unhealthy lifestyles such as nightlife, it has brought people a very serious consequence. 'Po' only performs detoxification at night while people sleep, but nightlife drinking resulting in being drunk every night has exhausted the defender 'Po' that guards our lives to the death.

Human organs all have spirits. In terms of body and spirit, the spirit is just as weighty and important. Proper daily life and diet can make acquiescent of blood and Qi to protect the body which results in unobstructed arteries and veins to gather Qi formation. Only the organ quality holds structure, only the power in the organ stores the spirit, to enable the blood and Qi to protect the body and allow the human to achieve the health.

If the diet is improper and unbalanced it will cause a lack of Qi in the body. When this occurs in female compatriots who allow the cold to invade their body, the result is infertility and dysmenorrheal due to cold uterus. This is not just a slight discord in the body. If one does not pay attention and continues to live such an unhealthy lifestyle, it will lead to a much more serious consequence.

The main cause of cancer is excessive consumption of cold food and sweets. Cold food, cold drinks, sweets, sugar, raw vegetables, frozen fruits and cold fruits etc. easily lead to cervical cancer, ovarian cancer, breast cancer and other foul diseases for women. Cold and sweet food easily brings dampness into the body.

Dessert especially can also make the stomach and spleen greasy. That is why people lose appetite after eating too many sweets. In other words, sweets harm the spleen and dampness is created when the spleen is hurt. Just as cold air drops (and heat rises), dampness will find the way downward and settle in the bladder, stomach and ovaries. Human weaknesses associated with this region of the body are most likely associated with dampness condition causing stasis. Malignant disease will outbreak when dampness has accumulated to a certain level over a long period of time. Therefore, ovarian tumors are a result of cold natured tumors. Hot natured tumors are easily found and diagnosed, but cold natured tumors are hard to spot. For example, if people enter an empty house they will feel and find the fire in the hearth as soon as they go in. This is determined by the radioactive nature of the fire. However, if the room instead were to contain a piece of ice, it would not be found so easily. Cold natured tumors harm the Yang. People who suffer from cold natured tumors hardly ever survive as the old saying goes, "Yang is long life". Over drinking of cold drinks, and grazing on sweets, sugar, cold drinks and frozen fruit are dangerous diet habits. Simply satisfying the taste regardless of physical ability to endure like this will inevitably lead to disaster.

Living with Taoism guidance

Here I repeatedly reiterate Taoist natural philosophy of life to make people understand the truth about the survival of mankind on earth as being inseparable from the values of Taoist Yin and Yang balance theory. Regardless of what advanced level the human technology has reached, led by today's capitalist development, it cannot get rid of the control of the forces of nature. That is, the more forward development of human technology, the more crises will be and the harder it will be to overcome; the more forward development, the more problems will be, and the more difficult it will be to resolve. Humans fall into a vicious circle which will see their demise in such a way. This is not sensational imagination; it is happening all the time in our lives but people just do not want to face it.

Humans now are simple and stupid like the ostrich in the desert who buries its head in the sand when in danger as if conditioned by a reflex with no account for a positive and effective defense. Humans are not ostriches, but the crown of creation and a most clever species with three spirits. So why have they returned back to the initial stage equal to the low level animal after a million years of long evolution and change? This has alerted us to review ourselves and recall what has resulted in a large degradation and setback of modern civilisation. The reason is that every time the human achieves revolutionary breakthrough in science and technology, they become alienated from the natural ecological balance by a mile. It is necessary for me to elaborate more details on this conclusion as to why every time the significant progress of technological revolution occurred; it has also caused great humanity retrogression itself. The reason for this is due to the nature of the scientific and technological revolution dictates. Unfortunately, on the other side of technological advance is a violation of natural law. The inherent human life and labor that includes mental and physical labor must not cross over the limit of natural law without the consequence of punishment. For example: before the car was invented, mankind depended on taming cows and riding horses to carry heavy weights and to move faraway by walking the complete trek. Thus people fully exercised their legs and limbs to give the body and brain natural harmony and development. This perfectly healthy body was not built from professional training at the gym, but from the labor of everyday life without paying any special attention. Neither did people have any expectation in advance as to what was required, but naturally obtained great results in terms of well-coordinated physical and mental health. This is just what happened unexpectedly and what arrived unexpectedly. People at that time simply did not know obesity and had no concept of diet broken down in terms of nutrition. This natural perfect healthy life came unstuck with the industrial revolution and mass-production of vehicles. The result was everyone had a car. People no longer lived a natural healthy way of life as they did in the past. Nowadays, people jump into the car and accelerate to the destination whenever they go out. Moreover, only one person enjoys driving a huge car in most of time. That is, not only does it pollute the environment but also creates a waste of resources.

Given a human is from nature, he should always abide by the principles and rules of the original life as it was when in harmony with nature, and therefore must not ignore the control of natural law due to his increased capacity. Otherwise, he will fall into the passive crisis and disadvantageous position. To understand the tightness of the relationship between human and nature from a deeper level, the important issue of how biochemistry in the universe is generated and changed needs to be considered. Like the relationship between the rise and fall of the moon and stars, the decrease and growth formatted Yin and Yang. This decrease and growth, rise and fall are inherent natural laws of Yin and Yang principles. It is associated with the formation and demise of all things and all matters. Nothing is separable from the general rule of the rise and fall of Yin and Yang. Its transportation mode specifically performs the four seasons and alternates rotation between day and night. Likewise, one year contains the cyclic seasonal rhythms, one day contains the diurnal rhythms. Just as the winter solstice marks the start of Yin, the summer solstice heralds the start of Yang, and a day's rhythm is the cyclic movement from Zi time (11pm-1am) to Hai time (9-11pm). The movement always in this cycle is unchanging since times immemorial. It is constantly repeated. Taoism calls this repeated life or usual change.

People live between the sky and earth, therefore there certainly exists a phenomenon between nature and human. That is, the Yin and Yang in the human body follows the rise and fall of the Yin and Yang of sky and earth to maintain people's normal life activities. Should this rule be violated when life is no longer routinely performed, such as not sleeping on time, or not eating on time, it will lead to disarray on the rise and fall of Yin and Yang and drive people to suffer various diseases. Therefore, the development that has broken humans away from the premise of natural laws can no longer be called development, but regression. In addition, we also face threats more dangerous than these bad habits and that is the arms race of mass destructive weapons. It captures human beings in a vicious circle from which they cannot extricate themselves. It engulfs the vast majority of human wealth and resources, and speeds towards destruction. The regretful and terrible thing is, thus far there has been no human force or effective way to stop the human community moving towards the destruction. To repeat mistakes like this over and over again puts us not far from the disaster.

Once you understood these principles can be used in practice as life guidance to get confirmation in life. But the general perception of today's people is to obstinately emulate the West. It is no wonder that more and more Chinese people today have no manners at all. They are further removed from the teachings of ancestors, becoming unworthy descendants who recount history but omit ancestry. A nationality that used to be in favor of morals has transformed and become villains seeking nothing but profit regardless of truth, morality, honesty and shame.

People are muddle-headed and chasing Western lifestyle. Much of society is sick and troubled. People don't stop and think if they support and accept gay and lesbian lifestyles, everyone may follow suit and become like that and then faced with no reproduction power, the society will end. People don't consider that the actions and beliefs they follow may result in dire consequence. This observation is not coming from a discriminatory point of view, but from knowing how change occurs and what evidently happens when Yin Yang balance is disrupted. If a man is no longer like a man, and a woman is no longer like a woman, the shameless man and the ruthless woman will become the portrayal of our 'new era'.

Taoist thoughts and academic treatises alike have

described thousands of years of life practices in China's long history as saving many innocent lives from falling into the line of death due to the chaos of war and extreme disaster. Throughout history, countless have been rescued across the entire country and nation. Therefore, today's descendants should not have the slightest inkling to doubt or distrust Taoism for any reason. The method for disease prevention and treatment has not changed and is fixed. But the theory is dialectical and flexible. Thus, the ideology and theory are the guiding keys to treatment through prevention.

Within one's lifetime, everyone goes through the birth, aging, illness and death. This is because all living things in the vulgar world cannot necessarily handle themselves on time when the opportunity arises, and therefore cannot necessarily keep the positive spirit inside. To relax ambition and reduce desire is to be content with ones lot and keep distance from lust as much as possible so one is not led to a fall through aging and sickness. Although a plant may deeply regret dropping its flowers, it should be noted that people do not die from age. That is, people do not die of old age. Rather, people die from disease. There is a reason we say the birth, aging and illness is followed by death, however as an interpreted truth from the other side "there is no separation of young and old in the underworld."

Taoist philosophy of a healthy way of life is to help people as much as possible to escape the cycle of birth and death. We have to start from the onset with a positive attitude towards following the requirements of a Taoist health regimen and be rid of bad habits in life. Habits include all aspects of daily life, such as the habits of eating, daily routine, work and exercise. Bad habits are those harmful to healthy habits. We have to make appropriate adjustments to let the good habits become the healthy regime. Certainly, this will require us to deeply study the ideology and theory with a willingness to achieve and make corrections. It may be necessary for us to list and name all the bad habits and symptoms in detail for the purpose of self-checking and self-restrain.

The most typical bad habit is overeating mostly due to eating disorders and impermanence. Not eating on time makes it easy to over eat because of too much hunger. Duration like this causes people to become overweight and unable to extricate themselves, catching them in a vicious circle. Once this bad eating habit is formed, it affects the people their whole lifetime. The first disease it brings to people is obesity, followed by a variety of sub-health symptoms or various diseases as a result. Moreover it makes self-image uncomfortable and embarrassing in public. The popular objective reflection and mental association with the obese patient is extremely negative. A reaction such as, these guys are short-lived or how much longer can this fat person live? Beautiful things like rainbows are never imagined!

In addition to over-eating disorders, other bad habits

such as drinking and smoking and addiction of various other kinds for example pharmaceutical drugs bring harm to health and life. Note, these poor eating habits can be changed. Like diseases, habits can be improved and cured over time through tireless effort or combined with some auxiliary force if required. Once changed, you will no longer be a slave to the habit and secondarily avoid the possibility of disease outbreak. We must first recognise the hazard of unhealthy habit and completely change it, and then combine some Taoist methods of self-cultivation to action change for the purpose of fundamental self-empowerment to become true masters of our own destiny.

The wisdom of Tao for the purpose of statecraft demonstrates positive life strategies for seeking opportunity and avoiding calamity. It is noted that everything in the universe has evolved from Yin and Yang. Yin and Yang are actually one with two sides of the same object. The two poles are connected and the relationship of exchange between the two ends, although opposite, remains united. To preserve long life we have to maintain the balance between Yin and Yang as much as possible. Balance is not a narrow performance emulating only one thing or one object, but an all-inclusive of all things and objects universally. In this context to follow the pulse of Taoist thought; we are able to reach the wonderland that connects humans to the sky, earth and positive spirits through the handling of

Yin Yang and good Feng Shui in daily life.

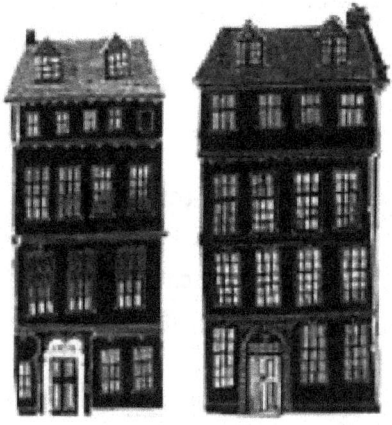

The arrangement of food and nutrition

For the purpose of health and life preservation, when we arrange daily diet, the first thing we need to take into account is the arrangement of the main staple food and non-staple food, and the arrangement of whole grains and refined grains. This will avoid many negative side effects that single nutrition brings to the body. Given modern people's diet structure is completely different from twenty or thirty years ago, food production has changed a lot. The nutritional balance and quality of food produced with the new technology has weakened a great deal, causing potential threat and harm to people's health. On the surface, today's market is booming and the era that marked not enough food and clothing has gone, replaced by the surplus and all the trouble that too complicated food has brought. When people fully enjoy the happiness of having ample food and clothing, new problems from time to time emerge into people's lives, making people confused, sometimes even miserable. The main manifestation is: unprecedented pressure of food production on farmers caused by annual population increase around the world. How to satisfy the growing population with the rising need for food? The answer is simple. That is to increase production of food. But there is no alternative way to solve the problem of food production except the extensive use of fertilisers and the technological age of genetic modification. As a result, it causes compaction of land, severe loss of fertile soil and extinction of harvest due to years of excessive fertiliser use. Excessive use of fertilisers and the technology of genetic modification also have a direct affect on the nutritional value of food resulting in grave side effects. These side effects will present in the future over a long time period as they continue to cycle, but one day when people are awakened to realise the harm, it will be too late. Considering the quality of the current food and the lack of nutrients and trace minerals, we should try hard to choose a variety of ingredients for cooking meals that have been produced by traditional methods to avoid cumulative damage to the body brought on by long-term eating of substandard food.

Below are several of my carefully selected simple homemade staple food recipes for readers and friends.

1. Beans and Rice porridge. Good to serve in winter months. Beans can be a variety of beans. Prepare after dinner by soaking rice and beans separately overnight. Cook the next morning by boiling.

2. Steam carbohydrate foods other than rice and wheat including sweet potato, yam and taro. The soluble fibre and bifid bacterium they contain can prevent colon cancer. The healthy cooking options are as porridge with

rice, steamed alone, or blended with flour to make bread. They are not good for frying as frying produces harmful carcinogenic substances due to the high temperature of oil.

3. Vegetable balls. Prepare 350 grams corn flour, 100 grams bean flour, 50 grams millet flour. Mix with boiled water to make dough. Cover and let stand for 10 minutes. Mix with chopped cabbage and separate into fist sized dough portions. Steam to cook then serve it.

Grain is the source of glucose. Carbohydrate of grains rapidly decomposes to glucose in the body which can cause an increase of blood sugar likely leading to hypertension and diabetes. The food that can elevate blood sugar fast is food with high glycemic index (GI); the food that can be digested easily is also food with high GI. The glycemic index of hard rice is low; the GI of soft rice is high. Refined wheat products such as hardened dry spaghetti, soft bread and noodles all have a high GI. The GI of unprocessed food is relatively low based on the high content of cereal fibre, but on the other hand processed foods such as crackers make blood sugar rise rapidly so the GI is high. Whole grains are low with GI; flour and rice are high with GI. Many people have misunderstandings about eating the staple food as they think the more white rice the better, and the more refined production the better. This is not right. It is necessary to always eat a little hard and unprocessed food and whole grains, and eat less soft, processed food and refined grains. By adding a portion of sticky rice whilst cooking a batch of rice, the GI will be reduced by 20% -30%. We should pay attention to arranging whole staple food with refined food enjoyed only on special occasions. To curb the sharp rise in blood sugar, aim for a slower release of glucose.

There is a very serious problem in current dietary trends (for example low carbohydrate, high protein diets) especially since people eat less and less staple food, and more and more animal meat. Animal meat is not healthy. The meat contains much higher oil than grain; for example duck meat contains 15% oil and pork contains as much as 30% oil. With the fat content three times higher than cereals, this makes it very hard to digest relatively. This diet structure of the new age threatens human health and is extremely serious and fatal. It can result in dyslipidemia that directly causes "big belly, long belt and short life". Therefore, people should strictly control their intake of meat, but not reduce the staple food.

Childhood obesity is another serious problem caused by eating; it should be adjusted in a timely manner. Elderly people should pay more attention to diet for health. "Skipping breakfast, lunch on the go, stodgy dinner" diet styles are all extremely dangerous. If these habits are not corrected in time, they will eventually lead to disaster.

In addition to emphasis on staple food in our daily

dining, we should also pay great attention to vegetables. Vegetables contain very low calories and are rich in a variety of indispensable elements such as antioxidants, fibre, minerals and vitamins beneficial to human health. It is an important part of a healthy regimen to choose vegetables that meet your taste and physical condition based on the characteristic of selected vegetables.

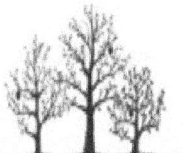

Prevention of excessive heat through diet conditioning

Previously cited are impacts and hazards of excessive heat (equivalent to fire), affecting people of all ages in the general society. Thus we have a better understanding of the excessive heat issue. Understanding though is far from enough; we should subject ourselves to more in-depth studies and research regarding ancient discussions on the excessive heat and experiences of dealing with excessive heat in the body.

Fire is a symbol of human civilisation. The universe is inseparable from the operation of fire. The collision of fire and water produces life, therefore fire is the source of life. Taoist theory of Yin and Yang talks about water and fire and the relationship between the elements. Water and fire are always inseparable. Yin exists where Yang is, Yang exists where Yin is. Yin and Yang can naturally find their own trajectory to achieve balance. Balance is eternal and is normal. Imbalance is momentary and abnormal. It is unusual to get excessive heat (equivalent to fire). Once the theory of Yin and Yang balance is understood, the true meaning and origin of 'excessive heat' will be figured out naturally. Therefore, this unusual state requires an effective balanced way to control the momentary abnormality.

Firstly, let's focus on how to cure 'excessive heat' varying from person to person. There are two types of people: 'fire' type and 'cold' type, which varies according to age, gender, geographical position, climatic environment and occupation. The treatment of 'excessive heat' is based on known guidance documents and is not to be compromised; otherwise it will cause side effects. The treatment of fire is akin to controlling with water, but the better rule with fire is to follow the direction it goes and assistance redirection by splitting it apart. In another words, to conquer fire is not just a matter of blindly throwing water, but to tactically divide and rule.

Medical theories originating in Taoism never paid attention to diseases that had already occurred, because preventative treatment was ingrained. The theory was not to rule disorders but to apply preventative measures in advance. To use medicine on already out broken disease is akin to ruling disorder after chaos as if unprepared seeking help at the last minute when already too late. Here, the ancients said, pay attention to preventative treatment rather than treating disease that has already occurred. This does not mean not to treat disease that has already occurred, but to emphasize prevention of the disease in the first place, thus actively adopting a prevention-oriented health care policy. Often people fall into a passive state, but should instead take the initiative. Lao Tzu said: "To relieve disaster or solve a problem is not as easy as prevention; to treat an illness is not better than to guard against it. People today are opposite and do not prevent it but treat it, and do not guard it but use medicine. Just as the monarch cannot always guard his country, people cannot always maintain the life. Therefore, the wise will seek happiness before the sign, extinguish disaster before the event. A disaster happens gradually whereas the disease grows slightly. People refuse to do even a small improvement as they think it is useless; people refuse to mend the way of small evil as they don't believe it to be destructive. Big virtue cannot be formed if small improvements are not accumulated; crime will be caused if small evil is not corrected." This text by Lao Tzu, the great Taoist founder, succinctly foretells true guidance as it relates to human existence.

Prevention-oriented health policy is not new for us. In the new China established since 1949, it seems we have been in unremitting practice for decades. It saved us a lot of additional cost in the era of the poor and weak. But when we entered the reform and open period, Western medicine in China expanded further. Since then, we no longer hear the voice of prevention. The reason is mainly because it runs counter to the theory and values of Western medicine; it significantly obstructs Western medical treatment for the purpose of making money. Therefore, in the era of reform and opening up, we no longer hear the prevention-oriented health policy. The contradiction we see between doctors and patients is growing more and more. Changes in health care policy make this great noble life-saving theory thrown beyond the highest heavens by the medical profession. This resulted in a very bizarre phenomenon of today whereby people go to the hospital for disease treatment. Not only does this not cure the disease, but it also makes people more and more sick from the treatment. The more disease you have, the more money it costs for treatment. No improvement can be seen from the treatment, but the money pocket is more and more flat. People are sent home to die when all the money is finally spent and nothing is left for treatment. This is still a better result compared to those who lost their lives because of misdiagnosis.

It should be heeded, there is no disease that cannot be cured in the world, there are only incurable people. If you are a Taoist, who is an honored practitioner following Taoist theory, you will never be at the core of passive struggle in life, you will always take the initiative for survival. Taoism advocates as long as you follow the Tao, enshrining the natural way, you will be able to handle the changing law of sky and earth of Yin and Yang, and then adjust the breath, take pure uprightness, consider self above worldly matter and live independently assured to keep the positive spirit inside. Exercise and slight labor of the body makes muscles and bones harmonised with the whole body to achieve coherency, so that life will endure as long as the world lasts. This is the result of Tao-cultivation and regimen. Otherwise, you will belong to a kind of incurable populous. When people suffer from disease unfortunately there is no Taoist guidance or knowledge to retrieve them from capture in the vicious circle of seeing the doctor again and again, treating again and again but not getting any better. This situation is very common today. This is because the opening up reform in China emphasizes Western materialism which inevitably leads to the imbalance dilemma of Yin and Yang in social life, based on hasty last-minute efforts. One-sided emphasis on the enjoyment of material things ignores the cultivation of positive spirit driving our modern society into 'civilised barbarism' unexpectedly. This so-called 'modern civilisation' is actually no better than the civilisation of savage 'barbarism'. At least the people of 'barbarism' are very pious and know how to follow the rules of nature without daring to show even a bit of frivolity. For example, a group of Tibetans drive yaks to travel and camp at high altitudes on an uninhabited region. Their purpose is to collect salt from the plateau salt lake. The tools they use are not of modern era. The hammer and club used for mining salt are made of horns. They eat in the wind; they sleep out in the snow. But they never forget to recite together their pious chant scriptures even under such harsh conditions. This is the mark of true human civilisation; this is the eternal portrayal in natural agreement with positive spirit. By contrast, 'civilised' people of today completely ignore the existence of an all mighty universal natural power, but rather do whatever they want in their own way. They are arrogant and uninhibited. They recklessly take rash action that may eventually lead all mankind to a big tragedy.

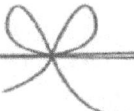

Conditioning diet to reduce the incidence of cancer

Experiments show that cancer and other tumor cells grow rapidly at low temperatures. That said, excessive cold natured vivo environments provide an opportunity for cancer cells to wantonly embezzle good healthy cells, and finally bring people to a tragic end. At present, three groups of the population are susceptible to gynecological cancer: the first group is the white-collar worker as the backbone of enterprise and elite across all walks of life; the second is the group of unmarried women with no children and no breast feeding; the third is the middle-aged people who are susceptible to various diseases due to decreased immunity during menopause and other so called troubled times.

The best way to treat cancer is the Chinese traditional fire needle acupuncture. Fire needle can build a defense against the invasion of unhealthy influences from the outside. The fire needle is used because the fire dispels the cold and needle removes the blood stasis. The fire needle is used to puncture and surround the part of human body with the cancer. Immediately after the fire needle is used to circumvent and perforate the area, 90% of people build an increased immunity. This is similar to the phenomena of inflammation when the skin is punctured by a thorn and the performance of the body's own immune system is activated. Cancer cell's worst fear is high temperature. The fire needle temperature is as high as a hundred degrees so immediately the cancer cells shrivel and die. In fact, no cancer cell can survive above forty-two degrees in any environment. Therefore, in avoiding cold foods and cold drinks, eating hot and cooked foods, taking hot drinks, keeping the body from getting cold and avoiding cold invasion into the body the incidence of cancer risk is effectively reduced.

There are many food therapies for cancer prevention. Ginger and black tea is one. The method is to brew black tea in boiled water with three slices of fresh ginger, and three grams of eaglewood powder. Eaglewood is known as the diamond of all plants, but eaglewood by nature is pure Yang so it easily makes excessive heat. It is better not to use too much eaglewood powder. Black tea enriches the blood and warms the stomach. Fresh ginger has the effect of warming the belly to fend off the cold. Combining these three can warm the stomach and protect the uterus. It is a good help for fixing cold and wet symptoms due to stagnation and poor circulation. Accordingly, due to the lack of Yang, hands and feet get cold.

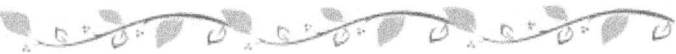

Conditioning five internal organs*¹⁶ through diet

Learning the basic functions and the role played by internal organs in the human body is elemental to the guidance of health regimen. The only way to keep the Yin and Yang balance of the internal organs is through the help of diet.

Liver is like the general officer; it plays the role of planning ahead in the body. Bile is like the honesty officer; it specifically makes a judgment and decision related to the human body. If a person is weak in the gall bladder, he will feel fearful, timid, indecisive, and lack decisiveness. Spleen and stomach are the warehouse management officers who accept and digest the food. The large intestine is the road for transmitting dross through the process of digestion, absorption and excretion. The function of the small intestine is to accept and hold down dietary reserves transferred from the stomach, it assumes the role of receiving and holding, and the task of digestion and absorption again. The dross is separated from here. Whilst the water partially penetrates into the bladder, the grain food dross moves down to the large intestine. Kidney can store original Jing (vital life fluid) and can create and nourish the bone marrow. The function of the kidney is to keep the body energetic, vigorous and strong. The role of the kidneys is strength. Lung dominates skin. Skin can drain moisture. Without the domination capability of the lung, a small lung capacity will lead to weakened lungs whereby people are likely to suffer from itchy lumps on skin, eczema and other diseases. If lungs are rich, skin will be moist and clear. Proper exercise can recuperate and enhance the lung capacity.

Human's evolution is based on different gender needs in the process of development. Men evolve physique and strong bones; women evolve reproductive function and store fat. Men are different from women in evolution, but neither can do without the adjustment of internal organs from a reasonable diet.

I have already presented several details on daily diet. The importance of which is how to use food to nourish internal organs; how to enrich blood vessels and empower positive spirit; and how to maintain a balance of Yin and Yang of internal organs to really achieve the purpose of health maintenance, extension of life and disease prevention.

To do this, we must master Yin and Yang properties of various food materials with the effect of Yin and Yang balance on internal organs. This is because when it comes to healthy regimen, the food has a most unique advantage. The advantage of diet is, without the negative side effect of toxicity, it provides miraculous results. Always consider the best choices when modulating disease. In the long history of China, the use of diet to adjust imbalances of Yin and Yang of internal organs can be said to be the main method of regulating healthy regimen and the most common prevention method of disease. In fact, to ensure Yin and Yang balance of the internal organs, the key is to health. But unfortunately, the whole world's people are currently lost in the morass of so-called civilisation of science and technology and unable to extricate themselves. Driven by rapid development in science and technology and huge economic interests, people easily marginalise or even abandon the traditional precious heritage of prevention and treatment of disease. This mankind who has forgotten themselves, due to the rapid development of science and technology of modern civilisation, has now fallen into a hopeless quagmire and is now even on the verge of destruction.

To get five internal organs healthy, you have to understand the effects of different foods in different seasons on the internal organs. More clearly, understand the relationship between diet and internal organs. What foods can help regulate the imbalance of Yin and Yang of the heart, and what foods can help Yin and Yang imbalanced lungs. What foods can effectively help the kidneys responding power, and what food can replenish the spleen and benefit the stomach? This book clearly informs the readers about each organ, allowing readers access to concise and practical knowledge to meet the needs of everyday life contingencies. Foods corresponding to the five internal organs, can directly impact on the health of internal organs, therefore this impact can directly affect a person's ability, emotion, intelligence and so on. Unfortunately, people often do not think about these issues beforehand as the bias thought process is to take common herbs to correct or adjust an imbalance of Yin and Yang and restore organ balance. Many people do not know that herbs have flaws because the accuracy of their dosage is difficult to master by the ordinary people. People trained in the use of herbs know to combine several herbs together and not to use one sort of herb on its own. As a result, the potency and efficacy of herbal medicine is difficult to monitor and it is not always known which herb or herbs played a decisive role in the end. There is a known saying that states Chinese medicine confusedly cures people for life, Western medicine clearly treats people for death. Therefore, taking into account all aspects of the use of herbs is not only difficult, but also requires the special needs of long-term accumulation of experience in order to achieve accurate prescription. The ordinary people cannot simply do this. However, for the ordinary people, treatment from diet is the best approach to health care. The majority of people are basically aware of the principles of food and the most preferable food that does not create side effects, unlike medicine. For example a person who is about to undergo surgery knows to eat less under modulation so as not to harm the life. The most ideal situation with food and Chinese medicine is that conceptually, it comes from the same source of good health care, in accordance with widely accepted knowledge adopted by social groups. This will undoubtedly help people in the world to improve and enhance the quality of their life; this will also provide nectar in a long drought for people who have fallen into a health crisis, with very positive and meaningful outcomes. I hope readers will clearly understand the special relationship between food and internal organs presented throughout this book, and adjust their own Yin Yang internal organ balance accordingly to maintain health.

Yin and Yang of the five internal organs is more directly affected by the environment, season, climate and diet. Although we cannot choose the factors of environment, season and climate, we can choose the factor of diet. If we can also choose food based on differences in our own physical condition, coupled with the geographical environment, season and climate, then we can really achieve good fortune and always maintain health.

To achieve timely diet, we must first make adjustments at the beginning of each season, however it is also extremely important to determine which of the four seasons marks the beginning of a seasonal diet. Should we follow the order from spring to winter; or the order from winter to autumn? To be clear about the sequential relationship, we must first understand Taoist fundamental theory. The sequential order is completely different from secular habits for which the order relies upon 'the end coming back to the beginning.' Taoists believe that the end of one cycle is the start. Emphasis is given to the topic covering 'order from end to beginning' on the matter of health regimen. It is related to the regeneration and storage of energy for growth; it can help people get proper nutrition into the body for the purpose of achieving health and longevity. Thus we determine the real beginning of the year starts in the winter months. Due to the special nature of winter, everything hides Yang energy deeply in order to meet the need for huge consumption of germination energy in the coming spring. If the energy cannot be hidden in winter, it means the germination in spring will not occur, and this in turn leads to no growth in summer and no harvest in autumn. No hibernation in winter will lead to the consequence of no energy for germination in spring. Thus we can understand the appropriate season to start the sequence for absolute safety, with twice the effect and half the effort.

Now, let us follow the order sequence from end to beginning to start the journey of full seasonal adjustment for balancing of five internal organs.

1. The conditioning of diet in winter
The Winter Chapter of The Great Account of Positive

Spirit Conditioning by Four Qi's in Yellow Emperor's Neijing Court Canon says: "Three months of winter is the season for hiding, lives submerge away, and all living things hide away. During this period, the weather is severe cold, the ground is frozen, and the earth is cracked in a pattern like the turtle's back. People should go to bed early in the evening and get up late in the morning. It would be better to wait for sunrise to get up. Disturbance of the Yang-Qi due to overwork must be avoided. People should often hide positive spirit deeply inside, as if a man does not dare show his secret to others; or as if to hide and hoard a treasure. To stay away from the cold and seek the warmth, and not expose the skin to the cold or to leak Yang-Qi are methods in line with winter weather for maintaining functionality hidden and stored in the body. If the Qi that should be hidden in winter is defied, it undoubtedly will damage the kidneys and make people suffer from fistula and fainting when spring comes, as the energy supply for spring germination will be affected."

The element associated with winter is water; it is an important season to nourish kidney but also the season sorely lacking in fire. Although lacking in fire, given winter belongs to the season of hiding and cold outside, internal heat is easily generated. In addition, not only is the internal heat easily generated due to outside cold, it can be traced back to the consequence of previous seasons during late summer and the beginning of autumn. In other words, the heat generated during the hot summer remains hidden in the human body before the advent of cold. The combining press of cold in late autumn and early winter cause heat energy to be trapped in the body. During the onset of autumn chill, it is better for people to wear less in autumn, thus avoiding too much heat remaining in the body that might cause the imbalance of Yin and Yang affecting winter's storage. Therefore we have to maintain the body's Yin and Yang balance during the winter hiding months, without interrupting internal heat. Too much heat will harm Yang and cause flu, damaging the root of the life which is considered a great taboo in the season of winter hiding. If accidentally attacked by excessive heat, mix kudzu (arrowroot) powder with hot water to immediately get rid of the heat and avoid Yang damage.

Winter is the season for preservation and nourishment. Due to the cold outside, in order to adapt to seasonal change, the human body naturally hides the vital kidney energy deeply inside to prevent leakage of kidney energy as much as possible. To ensure sufficient storage of energy and Yang-Qi to safely get through the long winter, and germinate vigorously with all living things at next spring return, we must follow the requirement of health regime in winter. Referred to herein as winter hiding, there will be nothing without hiding. During the so-called winter hiding, it is essential not to disturb Yang-Qi in the person's body. As the old saying goes, "nourish

Yang in winter, nourish Yin in summer". That is, as much as possible, do not engage in any hard activities in winter, keep nature moderated and calm, do not have excessively hot baths to avoid leakage of Yang-Qi but take winter tonic in accordance with specifics of the physical body of each person. Physically hot natured people should take cooling tonics, and physically weak and cold natured people should take more warm tonics. Winter is better for kidney nourishment so the people should eat more bitter and warm foods. Bitter and warm foods represent firmness and by draining out the diuretic dampness, kidney is strengthened and the body improved. The characteristic of bitter and warm natured food is Yin fire so it cannot burn out the kidney's Yin (the kidney liquid). Lamb is natured bitter and warm making it an ideal winter tonic to nourish kidney's Yin. People should not take too much tonic but follow the principle of "if there is an excess, then reduce it; if it is not enough, then replenish it", which is "the way of nature to reduce the extra and replenish the loss" although "the way of human" often is quite different, which is "to reduce the lack and increase the surplus". So "who does reduce the excess and replenish the loss in the world? Only the Tao."

If you do effectively save Yang and necessitate adequate nutrition for life in winter by appropriately maintaining balance of Yin and Yang, you will naturally lay a solid foundation for the next season's germination in spring.

2. The conditioning of diet in spring

The Spring Chapter of The Great Account of Positive Spirit Conditioning by Four Qi's in Yellow Emperor's Nei-jing Court Cannon says: "Three months in the spring season is called Fa-Chen, the growth; the natural world is in the thriving and vigorous germination and growth period. People in this time should sleep as soon as night falls and get up early in the morning and wear loose hair and clothing at the belt to relax the body as much as possible, enjoy walks in the courtyard to increase positive spirit and happiness. People should not wantonly kill creatures, should give away more and request less, should reward more and punish less. This is the way in line with Qi of spring germination. If the Qi of spring germination is defied, it will cause damage to the liver; make people suffer from cold natured disease when summer arrives and the energy supply in the season of long summer growth will be affected."

The element of spring is wood; it is the season to nourish liver. The human body begins to awaken after a long hiding in winter, and naturally acts to dry heat carried over from winter in the liver along with spring germinal forces, which leads to the moving up of liver heat. This is the typical phenomenon experienced that affects people's health and lives in the spring. Excessive Yang-Qi in liver directly induces liver-related diseases. If there is too much Yang-Qi in the liver, it cannot be adjusted by medication prescribed for liver directly, but relies upon the five elemental theories to adjust the balance of Yin and Yang of the liver. People should eat the food that can strengthen spleen appropriately which is sweet tasting food to complement and strengthen spleen. Earth natured spleen is strengthened, and earth can create healthy metal. If the metal is strong, it can naturally restrain excessive Yang-Qi of wood natured liver to make it balanced again. This is the ideal method of diet without side effect.

The point for regimen in spring is to eat sweet food to complement earth natured spleen and strengthen metal natured lungs to restrain wood natured liver to balance the excessive liver Yang-Qi in spring. Spring is the disease-prone season. The disease in spring is due to the liver problem and the liver is the Yang in Yin. The theory among Chinese medical treatments is not to treat the organ where the disease is, but to treat the related organ that causes the disease, to cure the source of that disease. This method of diagnosis and treatment is the unique concept of Chinese medicine theory. It is not only effective but also scientific. Sweet foods are our main source of nutrition. Sweet taste enters the earth natured spleen. Earth raises all living things. If you feel weak and need to complement, you should firstly look if you have eaten enough sweet property food which is the most important daily staple food, before rushing out to buy tonic. Sweet tasting food refers to staple foods such as rice and flour with a light taste. Rice, flour, sugar, freshwater fish, prawn, beef, corn and sweet potatoes are also sweet tasting foods. These foods play the role to complement the body and benefit the Qi, and to reconcile the spleen and stomach.

When choosing the food in spring, people should give consideration to foods that can nourish the spleen and stomach. Jujube, hawthorn and other sweet tasting food can be selected as preferred food in the springtime and can easily be absorbed by the spleen. These foods can help people to balance the internal organs, safely get through the spring, and keep the body in good condition for summer.

3.   The conditioning of diet in summer

The Summer Chapter of The Great Account of Positive Spirit Conditioning by Four Qi's in Yellow Emperor's Nei-jing Court Cannon says: "Three months in summer is the season with a mass of flowers and beautiful fruits. During this time, the atmosphere is moving down and ground energy is moving up, the energy of the sky and the energy of the earth intersect; plants are full of vitality, all living things are beginning to bear fruit. In this season, people should sleep later at night and get up early in the morning. People should not despair during long hot days, but maintain a happy mood; should not get angry, but raise their spirits to adapt to summer, venting unobstructed. To show an interest in external things like this is a release method in line with summer. If this is defied, it will cause damage to the heart and make people easily suffer from malaria when autumn arrives so that the energy supply in autumn harvest season will be affected and the state of illness will get worse in the winter."

The element of summer is fire; it is the season to support the growth. During the growth season in summer, the body has to get a lot of energy from the heart to meet the needs of summer growth, and then the heart has to get a lot of energy from the liver and kidney to sustain the growth. So people should pay attention not to make too vigorous heat in the heart. Too vigorous heat will harm lung's Yin. To calm the heart heat is to make kidney's Yin nourished. If kidney's Yin is enough, it will naturally calm the heart heat without making it too vigorous and thereby complying with the requirements of health for internal organs in summer.

To calm the heart heat, avoid giving medicine directly affecting the heart. People should specifically eat pungent foods to support and nourish gold natured lung to make more kidney water to balance heart heat. If kidney water is enough, it will be able to suppress the heart heat to prevent being too vigorous. This is the best way for heart adjustment in the months of summer.

4. The conditioning of diet in autumn
The Autumn Chapter of The Great Account of Positive Spirit Conditioning by Four Qi's in Yellow Emperor's Neijing Court Cannon says: "Three months of autumn is the

season of Rong Ping which is the peaceful and stable scene with mature vegetation and crops presented. The weather is clear and refreshing, the wind is strong, but the earth energy is cheerless during this season. People should sleep early and get up early synchronised with the rooster's routine in order to maintain the peace of mind to reduce the affect of cheerless autumn on the human. To moderate the spirit is to adapt to the climate of autumn and keep the body in a state of adduction for collection and nourishment during autumn. If this is defied, it will harm the lungs and cause suffering from diarrhea embolism and when winter arrives the energy supply for winter provision will be affected."

Autumn is gold natured; it is the season when lungs begin to converge descending, thus it is the convergence and regimen season. If lung is converged properly, it will provide people a smooth and safe transition from the bustling thriving summer to the cheerless melancholy autumn. This season is particularly difficult to unmarried marriageable men. As the old saying goes, woman feels sad in spring and man feels sad in autumn. That means it is easy to catch an emotional disease in autumn which makes people feel pessimistic and despaired in a bad mood.

In autumn, in order to dispel and dilute this sadness, it is necessary for people to find themselves as much happiness as possible to stabilise the mood from the sad of autumn. During the time of convergence and regimen in autumn, people should not forget to cultivate their own temperament and do as many activities as possible to benefit the health of their body and mind. The noble and elegant activities such as music, chess, poetry and painting are good choices for self-cultivation. These healthy activities can help people to restore innocence to perfect the spirit.

To achieve a converging regime in autumn, more sour foods should be considered as the choice for nursing liver and gall bladder. Acidity flavor is wood natured; it can easily be accepted by liver to support liver Yang. Liver is strong and can effectively help the heart heat; heart heat is strong and can suppress the lung's Yang so that the lung's energy will not be too strong to hurt the lung's Yin.

5. Five elemental chart

The so-called five elements are commonly known as wood, fire, soil, metal and water. The directions they represent are east, south, center, west and north; the seasons they represent are spring, summer, long summer, autumn and winter. The climates they represent are wind, heat, wet, dry and cold; The number they represent is eight. The order of the five elements to generate another is: wood generates fire, fire generates soil, soil generates gold and gold generates water. The orders of restraint are: wood restrains soil, soil restrains water, water restrains fire, fire restrains metal and metal restrains wood. The following chart shows in detail the relationship between the five elements.

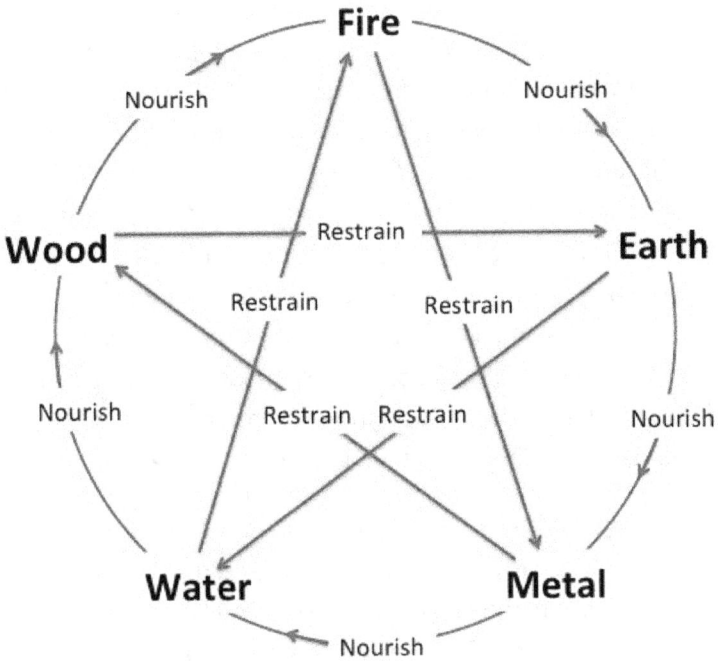

Eating for health

Examples enumerated in previous chapters are a true portrayal of today's life crisis. As though intimidated, people are not willing to face up to these truths. Most of these crises are caused by improper eating. The original meaning of diet was to maintain life, but today's meaning for diet has been transformed into main culprit harming people's health. This sounds a bit dumbfounding. In light of this, we should act now to bring back those precious Taoist theories about diet that have already been lost and restore them to take as a partner continuously leading us to eat for health.

Taoism is the Yin Yang theory about Yin and Yang's elimination and growth, rise and decline. The whole of existence in the universe is constantly changing in the form of Yin and Yang. At the moment when the universe initially formed from an unbound state, the heaven split and the earth was set apart. From one became two and this formed Tai Chi. Tai Chi is Liang Yi. Liang Yi is Yin and Yang, which is the original formation of the state of Yin and Yang, and as the sages said "Yin and Yang formed the Tao." Therefore, the universe is inseparable from the transformation and circulation back and forward of Yin and Yang. From this we understand that all things are controlled by the Yin and Yang. No matter what problem we encounter, we are supposed to follow the opportunity of Yin and Yang to adjust the Yin and Yang balance, to naturally restore the state that falls into a temporary disorder back to normal.

For daily diet and food therapy, we should pay special attention to observing and distinguishing Yin and Yang to verify comprehensively the particular Yin Yang properties for each particular type of food. To effectively target treatment for patients and prescribe with holistic diagnosis, we heed the problematic properties of Yin and Yang, the climatic geographical environment of Yin and Yang, and the characteristics of Yin and Yang in different people regarding gender and physical attribute. In summary, to utilise the Yin Yang property of food is to adjust body Yin Yang imbalances. Just as the sword is used to drive out the devil in Taoist Yin and Yang theory, we are able to overcome all the diseases and keep them away from us for good.

In daily life, we have to develop the natural balance of diet habits; we should always pay attention to adjust the Yin and Yang mix in diet and deeply understand the properties of various foods. We should replenish with some aphrodisiac food when the body is lacking Yang, and fix the deficiency of liver and kidney when the body is lacking Yin. We should identify two typical symptoms caused by the imbalance of Yin and Yang which are excessive heat due to the lack of Yin and weak heat due to the lack of Yang. In addition, we must uphold that 'food and medicine come from the same source' to achieve a sense of easiness in life. In the Chinese society we can say everybody knows the concept of 'food and medicine come from the same source'. Profound Chinese culture and thousands of years of life experience made it seared into the depths of the Chinese people's hearts. It is general knowledge in the guidance of daily lives rather than a popular folk saying. It informs a very important fact easily overlooked, and that is, the food itself is non-toxic and easy to control while the herbs are very different. The herb has a biased nature and is therefore difficult to be mastered and controlled in use. Especially due to the impacts of commercial tide, many sectors of herbal medicine planting, herbal medicine production companies and herbal medicine sales have experienced problems. The quality and right provenance of herbal material cannot be guaranteed, however this is precisely the crucial point for herbal medicine production. Not only is the quality of the herb important for pharmaceutical production, the efficacy of the medicine is determined by herbal origin provenance, the production season, the Yin or Yang of the land and ground level altitude. Chinese people have had a long history of being dependent on the collection of wild herbs. However, with the increase of population in today's society, coupled with the huge temptation of interest driven groups, the market has attracted unscrupulous businessmen, organising traditional

Chinese medicine in an extensive modern production way. The use of chemical additives is inevitable during any aspect of participation from the initial acquisition of raw materials to the finished product. As everyone knows, the medicine produced in this way not only makes loss of original efficacy and effect, but also harms human health and in severe cases even damages their lives. This is contrary to the fundamental concept of traditional Chinese medicine for life saving. Inevitably, chemical fertilisers and pesticides are used at the farm in planting herbal material for pharmaceutical production under the condition of modernisation. Resulting in an end product containing residual fertiliser and pesticide, these chemicals can block, slow down or even poison the purpose of the original medicine. That is why today's medicine efficacy is not only hopeless but harmful to people's life.

The true meaning of the sentence 'food and medicine come from the same source' is that it is close to the common people's daily life; it is as simple as the use of material and ingredients selected for cooking and tea brewing. The main purpose of 'food and medicine come from the same source' is to help people to relieve the suffering from illness not yet developed to a very serious disease. This option is the most ideal because it is non-toxic with no side effects. When a person has some minor illness, it may not be necessary to use a strong medicine for modulating, but instead eat some food to uphold and restore the body's balance of Yin and Yang in other ways. Food tonic is much better than medicine as every medicine has its poison. The poison referred to in Chinese medicine is not the poisonous toxic chemical contained in Western medicine, although this is truly hurtful to people and even causes death, but the poison of Chinese medicine refers to the deviation rather than the toxin.

To adhere to the theoretical guidance of eating for health, we must closely rely upon the simple thought of 'food and medicine come from the same source'. It is not from esoteric medical scriptures, but from humanitarian events nurtured by our unique country, unique cultural traditions and unique historical background. These naturally refined therapeutic practices and countless prescriptions are extremely consistent with everyday uses applied by the majority of the poor people. This knowledge among the people has been repeatedly used and confirmed in practice through many generations over the years. It is a full diet theory concluded through long-term continuous observations of the life. Although the region is wide, this does not block the therapeutic dissemination and diffusion throughout China from rural to urban areas, from the south to the north. History has proven that the Chinese nation has been more troubled than any other country across the world. The deficiency of doctors and medicine in the bygone era was the real disaster, with adversity and difficulty felt at large. In addition, China in that time was shrouded by years of war with people in dire straits. For survival, therapeutic prescription gradually brewed among the people was what came out of the hardship. If there was not the inspiration to create the wise Chinese medicine thought that 'food and medicine come from the same source', the Chinese nation would never have continued through numerous natural disasters. Just because of the simple and practical great realisation that 'food and medicine come from the same source,' it brought a glimmer of light in that long dark period to give people some consolation. Both historically and at present, people readily accept and learn the easy to operate 'business as usual' condition. Chinese people skillfully learn knowledge not by going to school and listening to the teacher but from experiencing the daily life. Most of them are influenced imperceptibly from an early age, and have naturally mastered a number of diet prescriptions from 'food and medicine come from the same source'. For example, people easily get faint due to heatstroke when working outdoors in a hot summer. In this case, to simply boil mung beans in a pot and make mung bean soup is an excellent medicine for the prevention of summer heatstroke. As another example, pseudo-ginseng is a very common herb in the southern part of China. Just the leaves saved many lives of people injured by weapons throughout the history of war in China. This diet prescription is now far reaching either side of the Yangtze River throughout cities and towns of

China. It can be smelled everywhere, is widely used and very effective. China is a worthy home of 'food and medicine come from the same source', being the birthplace of folk remedy and tested medical prescriptions for food as medicine.

In order to enable readers to understand the true meaning of 'food and medicine come from the same source', I have collected for readers some typical folk remedies and tested medical prescriptions that relate to 'food and medicine come from the same source,' and provided as an appendix. To keep it brief, I have only listed examples in part for readers to try as an entry-level learning. Despite the fact that some prescriptions may have omissions, they will still have the power to initiate effect. If readers feel there is still something more to learn, I will certainly increase descriptions in the next publication to accommodate.

People should maintain low-calorie and high-fibre in three meals every day. It is an unspoken rule of the basic daily diet to be followed. It is not necessary to be too rigidly adhering. It should be determined according to the different circumstances an individual may be facing. Principles of tonic taking and internal heat reduction of cause is substantially the same as the use of traditional Chinese medicine. The difference is the dosage is less precise. Because it is the diet, its bias is not as heavy as herbs, so more or less does not matter. Although it does not matter, it cannot be too much. It should not be overdone. No overdo no shortage. This is the way of diet. Therefore, if we can learn as much as possible from nature to ensure correct food and nutrition, with the Taoist theory to arm ourselves to regulate Yin and Yang balance, we will be able to keep away from disease, and return to health through eating.

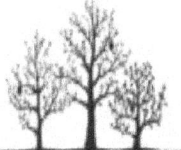

Taoist Diet Recipes and their effects

1. Ginger tea

Brown sugar with ginger as a tea in hot water can fend off the cold, treat stomach cold and prevent flu. To drink a cup of ginger and brown sugar after getting wet in the rain will help to sweat out the cold/ dampness from the body.

2. Chrysanthemum tea

Wild chrysanthemum has anti-inflammatory effects. To drink chrysanthemum tea may aid in the treatment of vaginitis and urethritis. To add chrysanthemum to the tub when having a bath can relieve eczema problems. Chrysanthemum is natured bitter and cold. It can easily harm the stomach. People with symptoms of spleen and stomach deficiency should be careful of this use.

3. Pineapple leaf tea

Pineapple leaves can sterilize and act as anti-inflammatory. Boil pineapple leaves in water and drink to treat diarrhea caused by eating unclean or stale meat.

4. Pseudo ginseng and fresh ginger tea

Pseudo ginseng and fresh ginger tea can improve blood circulation and nourish the blood. Angelica and rehmannia soup also plays a role in blood circulation improvement and has the effect of complementing without stagnation, supplementing deficiency and warming the body.

5. Hawthorn and rose tea

Hawthorn can eliminate retaining food in stomach, scatter bleeding and prevent cardiovascular disease; rose flower can smooth the Qi and eliminate depression, harmonise the blood and dispel blood stasis, improve blood circulation, detoxify and nourish the skin. If a person is not shiny but dark in face color and rough skinned, he must be in 'blood stasis' so he can take 30 grams of hawthorn and 20 grams of rose to make a hawthorn and rose tea for beauty, Qi and blood circulation, lowering blood pressure, smoothing liver Qi, reducing stagnation and improving digestion via stasis removal.

6. Bergamot and ginger tea

Bergamot has effects to rectify Qi and transform phlegm, stop vomiting and eliminate gas, smooth liver, strengthen spleen and comfort stomach. It can also reduce heat to relieve bronchitis and asthma in the elderly. For others it can treat indigestion and distension of chest and stomach. Add bergamot and rose to boiling water to make bergamot rose tea. Alternatively boil or brew bergamot with ginger to drink as tea.

7. Orange peel tea and orange seed powder

Orange is sweet and sour tasting, and cool natured; it has effects to help thirst, appetite and carry down the gas. Orange is full of treasures. Orange flesh can stop vomiting and nausea, and detoxify fish and crab. The orange peel can return appetite and comfort stomach; orange seeds can cure hernia and lumbago. To soak orange peel in water for drinking can help digestion and eliminate phlegm. Also this water can be used to wash hair and face leading to the conditioning of hair and beauty. By boiling orange peel and winter melon peel together with sugar for drinking as a tea, one can benefit diuresis, dispel phlegm and heal any swelling. To ground dried baked orange seed into powder, take and put 3-5 grams into boiled water and drink it after meals. It can treat rheumatism to a certain level with long-term adherence. To eat orange with white wine can cure acute twisted back and eliminate back pain.

8. Lotus juice

Lotus is cold natured with both a heating and cooling effect. It can be used to treat heat related illness. Use 500 grams of raw lotus root to make juice for the purpose of cancelling liver heat.

9. Fruit and veggie juice

The fruit and vegetable drink made of a mixture of pears, lotus root, phragmites root and fresh water chestnuts is sweet tasting and cold natured. It has a stomach nourishing effect. It can be used to reduce stomach heat. It is a good dose of food as medicine to comfort spleen and stomach, and a good drink to nourish stomach.

10. Lamb and Sugar Cane Soup

Lamb is a warm natured food. It can supplement Qi and nourish Yin, warm up the body and help the weak, create appetite and strengthen power. The Compendium of Medical Herbs calls it a warm tonic that fills Yang energy and benefits blood and Qi. Sugar cane is a food that cools down the body and reduces excessive heat. To cook in a soup both lamb and sugar cane provides the perfect contraindication solution for people who easily get excessive heat when having tonic food caused by prosperous heat due to the lack of Yin. By supplementing the nutrition from lamb meat and using sugar cane's heat removal function to balance the heat of the lamb it treats and conditions the people with prosperous heat due to lack of Yin. Lamb stew with yam and potatoes can be a winter tonic to nourish Yin and strengthen Yang. However, the following should be noted when consuming lamb meat: a) people with symptoms of fever, toothache, mouth sores should eat less; b) people with high blood pressure, liver disease, acute enteritis or other infectious diseases should eat less or not eat at all; and c) it is not advisable to drink tea right after eating lamb as it will lead to defecation or constipation.

11. White hyacinth bean soup

White hyacinth beans have effects that benefit and nourish the lungs. Boil white hyacinth beans, cogon grass root, phragmites root and red beans together to make a soup for drinking that can nourish lungs and prevent lung disease. In accordance with the season and the physical condition of the body, the drink can be made with slight derivation by using white hyacinth beans and mung beans to restore balance to the body. This can effectively clear the heat, detoxify and prevent flu. The prominent feature of this prescription is low-calories and high-fibre. It is the ideal drink for health conditioning.

12. Loofah peel soup

The loofah peel can calm kidney heat. Drink loofah peel boiled soup can help the treatment of prostatitis and heart disease caused by excessive kidney fire.

13. Pseudo ginseng, angelica with black chicken soup

Angelica has an effect on blood supplementation and blood circulation improvement; pseudo ginseng is also the first medicine to supplement blood. Pseudo ginseng, angelica with black chicken soup can help condition a physically congested body.

14. Soft-shelled turtle and lamb soup

Soft-shelled turtle has the effect of cooling the blood which is detoxification. Soft-shelled turtle and lamb soup can nourish Yin, refill spirit and cool blood. Taken as a winter tonic food it can warm up the body and feet, nourish Yin and comfort the stomach. It can help with symptoms of dizziness and tinnitus due to the deficiency of kidney's Yin and the lack of spleen and stomach's Yang. Hot flushes, night sweats, internal stomach cavity and abdominal pain, cold and poor appetite can all be improved. But people with too much moisture in the body are not suited for consumption of turtle.

15. Sugarcane and yam soup

Sugarcane is flat natured and can enter lungs; it has nourishing and moistening effects. Sugarcane is rich in amino acids and trace elements the human body needs such as calcium, iron, phosphorus, manganese and zinc. The body can easily absorb the sucrose, glucose and fructose it contains. Sugarcane and yam soup can cure cough; sugarcane skin and wheat porridge can cure sweating and help strengthen a weak heart.

16. Pigeon soup

The pigeon meat is salty tasting and flat natured; it has effects to nourish the liver and kidney, it can strengthen the body, clear the lungs and smooth circulation. Pigeon soup can warm the internal organs of the heart, lung, kidney, liver and spleen. It is especially good for people with weak kidney to consume and for children who are distraught and growing.

17. Rice and astragalus porridge

Astragalus has effects to supplement Qi and sharpen appearance, stop perspiration and detoxify. Also acts as diuretic and eliminates swelling. Astragalus porridge is most suitable for Qi supplementation; it can promote metabolism and therefore play a role in weight loss. It also can treat constipation caused by the lack of Qi. By cooking rice and astragalus porridge in summer, nutrition largely lost from the human body due to sweating can be supplemented.

18. Skinned peanuts and rice porridge

Peanut has effects to supplement blood and nourish lungs. Skinned peanuts and rice porridge can nourish the Qi in blood and intestines, and moisturize the skin for beauty. It is suitable for consumption by anemia patients, people with rough skin prone to dryness and people with habitual constipation.

19. Citrus and rice porridge

Citrus can rectify Qi and strengthen spleen; it has effects to drive away dampness and dispel phlegm. It has a good therapeutic effect on bloating, belching, loss of appetite, indigestion, chest diaphragm stuffiness, nausea, vomiting, cough and phlegm. In the season of autumn and winter, people easily get internal heat and phlegm; people are also susceptible to flu and cough. Citrus and rice porridge can dispel cold, rectify Qi and soothe the nerves. It is most suitable for people to consume for the purpose of maintaining health in autumn and winter.

20. Millet porridge

Millet is sweet and salty tasting with cold nature; it is also rich in phosphorus. It can nourish the heart and calm the mind to help improve sleep. It can also nourish stomach, comfort stomach and clear stomach heat. Boil the water and roughly washed millet then cook for 45 minutes to make porridge. To eat millet porridge in the evening is most helpful for calming the mind, nourishing Yin and blood, and strengthening spleen and stomach.

21. Rice and mint leaf porridge

Mint leaves are spicy tasting and cool natured; it has effects for evacuation of wind-heat, smoothing the liver, improving circulation, clearing the mind and clearing the eyes. By cooking rice porridge with mint you can improve nasal cavity function. It has good supplementary effects for the treatment of runny nose, rhinitis and migraine.

22. Rice vinegar soaked radish

Vinegar has many functions such as blood circulation improvement, bleeding staunch, detoxification, killing germs, deworming, appetizing, softening blood vessels, lowering blood lipids and improving metabolism. Vinegar soaked white radish can soften blood vessels, help treat atherosclerosis, blood pressure and govern internal disease from outside. To mix schisandra (Wu-wei-zi) with vinegar can benefit Qi and nourish Yin. It acts as antiperspirant to stop diarrhea and improve metabolism. It can assist in the treatment of premature ejaculation, nocturia and prostate enlargement. It can also stop children's nosebleed.

23. Boiled Duck eggs and duck eggs fry

Duck is cold natured; it can clear lung's heat. Salt taste can enter the kidney. Salted duck egg has the best effect for clearing heat. It also has conditioning effect for cough and eczema. The most common way is to boil salted duck eggs and eat with porridge. Alternatively, fry beaten raw duck eggs, after ginger powder and salt have been stirred in as for ordinary methods of egg scramble. If you add a little vinegar, it will taste delicious like crab meat.

24. Red bean buns

Red beans have the effect of nourishing the heart, supplementing blood, replenishing Qi, making the heart tissue unified, settling the positive spirit, calming nerves and more. Most Chinese Northerners like to use red bean paste to make red bean buns to eat.

25. Rice vinegar soaked black beans

Black beans have specific effects that benefit liver and kidney, and nourish stomach. There is a known proverb among the people "To live long, eat black beans". By soaking baked black beans in vinegar you can supplement kidney strength resulting in weight loss, bright eyes, blackened hair, white face skin and anti-aging benefits. Long-term eating of vinegar soaked black beans can prolong the life.

26. Yam and wolfberry beef stew

Yam supplements the Qi, wolfberry benefits kidney and liver. Beef stew with yam and wolfberry can supplement Qi and benefit kidney, strengthen bones and muscles. It is good for people with liver and kidney deficiency to consume. Sore back and knee pain due to osteoporosis can also be improved.

27. Roasted or stewed prawn

Prawn is high in nutritional value. It can enhance the body's immunity and sexual function; it can supplement kidney and strengthen yang and it can prevent premature aging. Eat fried, roasted or stewed prawn regularly with warm wine to cure impotence caused by weak kidney, prone to cold, body tiredness, back pain, knee pain and other symptoms. If suffering symptoms of postpartum, take less milk or no dairy at all. Finely chop 500 grams of prawn meat, cook and eat with hot yellow wine three times a day for a few days. This can effectively play the role of prolactin. Small dried shrimp has the function of a sedative which is suitable for warming and Yang supplementation. It can be used for the treatment of neurasthenia, autonomic dysfunction embolism and supplement calcium.

28. Seaweed and meat stew or sweet and sour seaweed stir fly

Seaweed is rich in trace elements beneficial to the human body, such as iodine, calcium, sulfur, iron, sodium, potassium, magnesium, cobalt, phosphorus, mannitol, vitamin B1, etc. The mannitol it contains can lower blood pressure, act as diuretic and eliminate swelling. Seaweed can cure liver, stomach and kidney disease; it can aid against inflammation, cure lymph nodes and goiter, treat edema, and treat difficult urination; it also can inhibit hyperplasia. In addition, seaweed has a conditioning effect on hair. Regular eating of seaweed can prevent cardiovascular disease. Stewed meat with seaweed, or sweet and sour seaweed stir fly are all good diet recipes.

29. Shepherd's purse soup and dumpling

Shepherd's purse is known as a wild vegetable. Spring shepherd's purse can dispel cold and reduce heat. Shepherd's purse picked in early spring has best efficacy. Forage some from outside the city to make soup, or cook with other foods such as eggs and seaweed together for a tasty and delicious soup. For an even more miraculous effect, chop shepherd's purse to mix with mince to make a filling for dumplings.

30. Bok choy root shampoo

Bok choy is rich in calcium and phosphorus with a high nutritional value. It has supplementary effects for skin care and breast cancer treatment. Bok choy root is rich in crude fibre; it can ease constipation and promote detoxification. It also has a good effect on the prevention of colorectal cancer. To boil bok choy root and use the water as shampoo can prevent hair loss; to boil bok choy with brown sugar and fresh ginger for drinking hot can cure the flu.

----------- ⋅ E N D ⋅ -------------

Dongyang

Foot Note

*1 Taibai mountain: Taibai Mountain is located on the border between Mei, Taibai and Zhouzhi Counties in the south west of Shaanxi Province, China.

*2 Sun Simiao: The great Taoist master and famous traditional Chinese medicine doctor of Sui and Tang dynasties.

*3 Qi: The original energy in the blood.

*4 Yin: The Taoist concept of nature as viewed by ancient Taoists who found out the truth of natural phenomenon and the mode of relative existence. Yin is the negative part of nature such as earth, moon, night, cold, female, down and so on.

*5 Yang: The opposite of Yin. Yang is the positive part of nature such as sky, sun, day, hot, male, up and so on.

*6 Five elements: The five elemental theory is about the basic elements in nature, including metal, wood, water, fire and earth.

*7 Ying-Qi: The negative energy. When the negative energy level rises high, it will bring the illness and a bad mood such as depression and so on.

*8 Yang-Qi: The positive energy. When the positive energy is dominant, it will manifest as happiness and health both mentally and physically.

*9 Ren-Mai channel: Conception vessel. Although called the conception vessel (Ren-Mai channel), this extraordinary meridian is much more than just the power behind reproduction.

*10 Chong-Mai channel: One of the eight veins on the human body. Documented in "Su-wen, the bone theory" and other traditional Chinese medicine books, the pulse can regulate the blood through twelve channels known as the twelve meridians of the sea. Functionality of the reproductive system is closely related to meridian function. If a woman's Ren-Mai pulse is strong, her excretion of menstruation will be normal. That's why Ren-Mai channel is also known as Blood Sea.

*11 Dai-Mai channel: The belt channel is one of the eight channels or veins. Dai-Mai can constrain the longitudinal line of the pulse. Foot San-yin, Foot San-yang, Yin stuck and Yang stuck pulses are all subject to the constraints of the Dai-Mai pulse to strengthen the link between the meridians. Dai-Mai channel's main division of the role is the protection of the fetus and the women. Dai-Mai channel line starts from the side abdomen, runs obliquely down to the Dai-Mai pulse around the body and then goes along the upper edge of the hip to the belly.

*12 Huo-luo-dan: A medicine elixir pill for treating stroke.

*13 Excessive heat: Known as Shang-huo in Chinese, excessive heat can have several symptoms, which are generally connected to a sense of inflammation. It is characterised as redness on the face, swelling, fever, and pain. However acne, sore throat, nosebleed, skin rashes, swollen gums and canker sores are also symptoms connected to excessive heat.

*14 Jing: The body liquid of human and the basic form of life such as sperm and blood.

*15 Shen: The positive spirit which is a combination of Jing and Qi to make a life. Jing, Qi and Shen are the three basic energies of human life.

*16 Five internal organs: The five elements in nature are reflected in the human body as five internal organs including heart, spleen, lungs, kidney and liver. The five organ system is the main Chinese medicine theory for treatment.

Dongyang

Postscript

Today, very few people can consciously reflect on exactly what's missing from today's lifestyle compared with previous years. If anyone can jump out of this circle to look at today's world from a spectator's perspective with historical macro point of view, he will be stunned by what he sees.

Because of the revolutionary force of productivity increase, a fundamental change in lifestyle and values has resulted. This change has affected all aspects of social life. Only during the development and change in this short period of recent decades, have people instantly erased historical memories of many generations without leaving any trace. People today have suddenly lost the past almost overnight, and loss of the past will also result in loss of the future. It is easier to forget history than to bear it in mind. However, forgetting the past also means lost future. Therefore, we must spare no effort to seize the past and not let it slip away or drain from our memory. We must mine the past to awaken the sleeping spirit in order to truly perceive the future and then to face and have a future.

We should have an objective and clear understanding of human development today so that we don't doubt all those precious health regimen writings that ancestors left for us. Don't let this abandonment happen because of the so-called great progress of medical technology today. There are contemptuous people who disdain the popular prescription of diet as beneath them, who narrowly think today's science and technology should dominate humanity, who no longer need traditional healing methods and deem such concepts as 'witchcraft' or 'superstition'. Actually, this thought process is bound to cause periodisation and loss of too much precious heritage. In addition to the Chinese medicine saving lives of people suffering, there are also recipes of 'food and medicine come from the same source' in these precious heritages. These recipes are more easily acceptable by the majority of ordinary people. It is an extremely important landmark to inherit and carry forward these great national treasures.

The Chinese nation has never had a shortage of massive historical heritage. It is because we have gone through long and winding roads more than any other nation. There was sorrow, there was joy, there was sinking, there was brilliance. Along the way, we have in one hand carried a heavy historical burden, and in the other hand held the key to a brighter future. History makes us mature in the next moment so let us forge ahead and own the link to connect past and future.

Tao and Diet

ABOUT THE AUTHOR

Master Dongyang started learning at a very early age in Beijing, China. His teacher is Wang Mingli who came form Zhongnan mountain, where the genuine Taoist lineage established.

From the very start, Master Dongyang learnt genuine Taoist knowledge, which is non-superstitious and non-religious but true natural knowledge and natural practice to cultivate and grow the internal elixir (Neidan)

Branched out from Taoist lineages that stemmed from private Taoist hermits, Master Dongyang promoted Tao as a practical, effective and functional way to easily deal with variety of troubles and issues. There are no rituals and rites, there are no chants or prayers. There is only a simple life cultivation through the cultivation of the internal elixir and the constant respect of the nature.

Master Dongyang is constantly doing hard to bridge the gap between the ancient Taoist knowledge and the modern world to spread the Taoist theory of the life to public through his Laozi Academy in Sydney, Australia.

Now, Master Dongyang is trying to use easy to understand language in this book to share his Taoist knowledge to more people who is keen to learn about Taoist knowledge. He hope his readers can be benefit from this book.

Tao and Diet